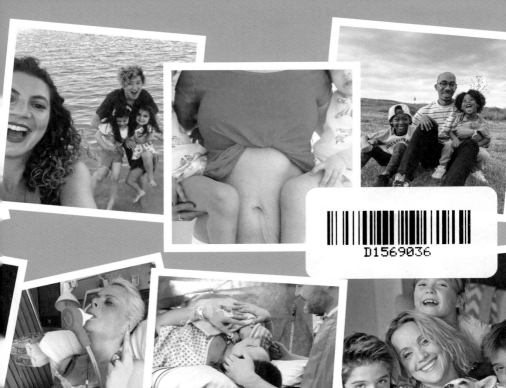
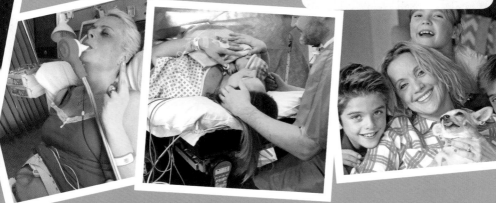
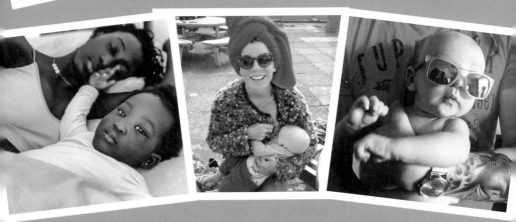

D1569036

Nobody Tells You . . .

OVER 100 HONEST STORIES
ABOUT PREGNANCY, BIRTH
AND PARENTHOOD

Becca Maberly

with expert advice from Roger Marwood
MB BS, MSc, FRCOG

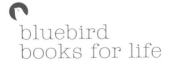

bluebird
books for life

To my husband Tom – without you, I would
never have written this book.

To my sons, Wilfred and Gus – without you, I could
have written this book much more quickly.

I love you dudes.

Contents

About the authors

—— BECCA MABERLY

Becca is the eldest daughter of obstetrician and gynaecologist Roger Marwood, and has become a pregnancy and postnatal expert almost by osmosis. She is the founder of A Mother Place, which offers online antenatal classes and support for the postnatal period. She is also the mastermind behind The Doctor and Daughter Antenatal Classes, which have been running in London since 2014.

When pregnant with her first son she was shocked by the lack of honest and reliable information available. She undertook to learn as much as someone can about pregnancy and birth without actually going to medical school and then bullied her father into starting the website and the classes with her as she was convinced that they could do better than the traditional offerings.

Having an obstetrician father at the end of the phone means that she has access to the very best information 24-7. This is a huge privilege which she has always wanted to share with as many people as possible – just ask her friends, many of whom have had Roger on speed dial throughout their reproductive years!

Becca lives in South West London with her husband and her two boys, and loves spending time with them and swimming . . . but not at the same time!

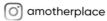 amotherplace   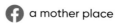 a mother place   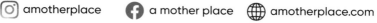 amotherplace.com

ROGER MARWOOD

Mr Roger Marwood MB BS, MSc, FRCOG is a recently retired consultant obstetrician and gynaecologist who has more than 40 years' experience of working in a busy NHS hospital and has personally delivered more than 5,000 babies. He has also supervised approximately another 20,000 births.

Although a lifetime supporter of natural childbirth, Roger believes that with proper and honest antenatal education, appropriate interventions in the delivery room can be part of a fulfilling and amazing experience.

As a gynaecologist, he is aware of the unique role played by the pelvic floor, and the importance of reducing trauma and preserving function. He has also been a longstanding pioneer of the "gentle caesarean section".

He is a past president of the Obstetric and Gynaecology Section of the Royal Society of Medicine.

For the last 20 years he has been a senior lecturer at Imperial College of Medicine, where he has been an acclaimed and popular teacher and tutor.

He has worked extensively for the Royal College of Obstetricians and Gynaecologists, and is currently one of their media spokespersons.

Roger is a father of three and dabda (grandfather) to five. He enjoys sailing, sculpting and swimming.

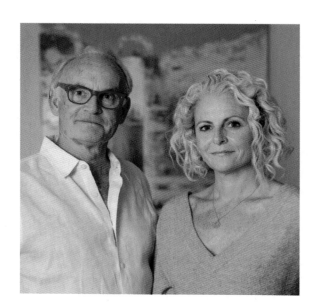

Roger Marwood & Becca Maberly

Introduction

My pregnancies were pretty "textbook", apart from some bleeding (terrifying) and my births were better than I could have imagined (quick and in a birthing pool), but before you write me off as smug, what came next was a huge shock to me. I found the postnatal period so difficult. The physical side of becoming a mother had not fazed me at all, but the emotional side completely overwhelmed me. I struggled to adapt to my new role in life and to accept my "new normal" and was ashamed to admit to anyone that I was not particularly enamoured with the whole "motherhood" thing! Breastfeeding was an unexpected struggle and sleep did not come to us like the books said it would.

My expectations were so out of line with the reality and this made me mad! There seemed to have been so many details shrouded in secrecy – insider information, to which you were only allowed access after having your baby. I was angry with my friends, my own mother, the books and the classes for failing to tell me what it was really like and not giving me the information I needed to prepare properly for the most momentous time of my life.

My frustration at the lack of honest and reliable information available, has, since then, driven my passion to educate the new mums and dads coming behind us. I want everyone to know what it is really like to be a new mum or dad . . . but not just based on my experience, as I am only one of the thousands of women who give birth every day.

Some of you will sail through parts of pregnancy, birth and parenthood, some of you will struggle, but most of you will have a mixture of remarkable experiences and challenging phases, with some shit-shows thrown in for good measure. There will be times where you feel like you're nailing it and other times where you feel like you can't go on, but you can. And you will. We hope this book helps.

Becca x

—— CONTENTS

Getting pregnant

Getting pregnant is not always as straightforward as we might expect. For some women and their partners this can come as a real shock. But everyone's experience is different, which is why it can help to hear about others in the same situation as you.

This chapter offers support for those who are just starting out on the path to parenthood and highlights some of the stories that Nobody Tells You . . .

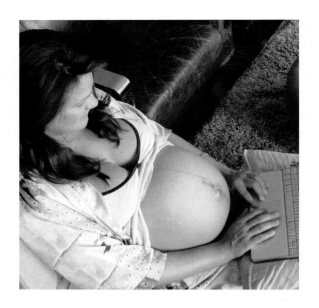

Sometimes it happens quickly!

Izzy Ansell @thisisizzyansell

I'm embarrassed to say those school biology lessons clearly hadn't registered for me! I had come off the pill before we got married to give my body a break rather than to get pregnant . . . I just assumed it took ages and we would "try" (awful expression!) at some point that year when we were "ready".

I had absolutely no idea what ovulation was or when it was and I barely knew what was going on with my own cycle having been on the pill for years.

I'll never forget being at work one day and suddenly realising

I had sore boobs but hadn't had a period for ages . . . oh . . . I think I could be pregnant . . . duh! It happened straight away.

It was quite a shock and I remember being really worried about how work would react. I was very nervous about becoming a mum but it all worked out beautifully in the end.

Looking back it was such a lovely and exciting way to get pregnant: stress free, lots of fun, no peeing on sticks or counting days . . . Baby no. 2 was not so easy, but that's another story!

—— OUR ADVICE

Absolutely no one will be able to tell you exactly when you will get pregnant. There are so many factors at play, including your age, your health, the quality and quantity of your eggs and your partner's sperm.

Although we have all heard stories of couples for whom trying to conceive is a difficult and lengthy process, you should not be too surprised if it happens quickly for you: 30% of couples trying to conceive will get pregnant in the first month. This can feel like a bit of a shock, especially if you weren't sure you were ready and if you and your partner were looking forward to the "trying" part!

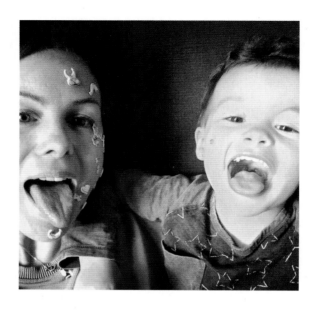

Sometimes it takes longer than you hoped

Suky Arneaud @the_ivf_mum

Nobody tells you that it could take four years, seven rounds of IVF, five missed miscarriages and many highs and lows to create my beautiful son. Would I do it again? Yes, 100%. He is worth all of those struggles and that long journey. It means I'm a little bit older than I hoped to be as a mother of a toddler, but that really doesn't matter.

Nobody tells you that male infertility sometimes needs to be looked into properly and that pushing a couple straight into IVF is not always a good idea and can lead to heartbreak that could have been avoided.

Nobody told me that I had a rare blood group until three rounds in, or that my own immune system could be fighting against our embryos. I wish I'd known all that I do now at the start of our journey, but the journey made our relationship stronger and we got there in the end.

And guess what? We did it again and now I'm almost 17 weeks pregnant with my second baby, and it happened first time this time and I still can't believe it!

—— OUR ADVICE

If you have spent the majority of your fertile life trying to avoid getting pregnant, you may be shocked to find out that once you actually start trying to make a baby, it does not always happen as quickly as you might hope and sometimes you may need help to conceive.

Both men and women can suffer from fertility issues, and these can be as a result of age, weight, sexually transmitted infections, smoking, alcohol, environmental issues and stress.

Sometimes the problem is with the woman's eggs, fallopian tubes or lining of the womb, and sometimes it can be the quality of the man's sperm. And sometimes no obvious cause can be found.

IT IS A GOOD IDEA TO TALK TO YOUR GP IF:
• you've been trying for a year and haven't conceived
• you are over 35 and have been trying for six months
• you have any reasons to be concerned about your or your partner's fertility

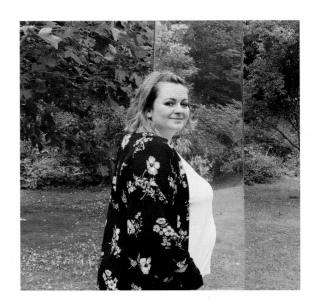

When the time is right

Amy Gorse @birdgurl_28

On 22 November, I did a pregnancy test, purely to rule out the unlikely possibility I might be pregnant. It was positive. I was in complete shock – for someone who'd never wanted kids, this completely caught me off guard. My first thoughts were panic, even more nausea, my relationship, my independence, money and ultimately whether abortion was the best option.

Suddenly I found myself thinking about a cute baby, with my eyes, and my whole attitude changed. This was something I was getting excited about, and that excitement grew over the next month. Then came one of the worst days of my life. The 12-week scan that told me, after falling in love with something I'd never known I wanted, I'd lost it. It's a day that led to surgery on Christmas Eve for surgical management of a miscarriage. But, it's a day that showed me exactly what I wanted. After 27 years, I knew what I wanted so much it hurt.

Fast forward and I am now extremely fortunate to be sitting here nearly a year later, 31 weeks pregnant and eagerly awaiting the arrival of my little girl just before Christmas.

—— OUR ADVICE

There is no right or wrong time to start trying for a baby. For some women the decision is more practical, based on consideration of finances, careers, number of bedrooms or stage of life. For others the decision is more emotional and is the culmination of a lifetime of broodiness, a desire to become a mother, a yearning to procreate with a partner, the need to fill a gap or the desire to create new life as another life finishes elsewhere. And sometimes . . . it just happens! For most women it is a mixture of the emotional and practical, and like many monumental decisions in life there is often much deliberation and uncertainty to overcome before deciding whether or not you're going to go for it!

Sometimes you just have to take a leap of faith. If you decide that you are going to go for it, then good luck and make sure you are eating a healthy and balanced diet, not smoking or drinking alcohol and start taking your folic acid before you even start trying! If you have any medical issues or are on any medication please speak to your doctor first.

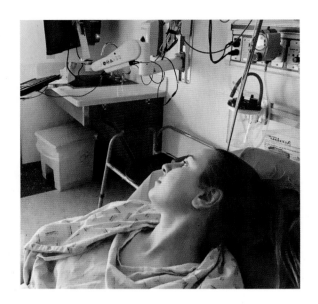

Miscarriages are more common than you think

Laura Abarbanell @tough_cookie_laura

It all happened so quickly. After our wedding we decided that we would just start trying and whenever it happens, it happens. I got pregnant straight away. Whoa! That fast? Are we ready? AM I READY?

We told our families and close friends and were showered with so much love and happiness from them. Those were precious moments of happiness when I didn't worry about anything. We were going to have our first baby!

Week 6 – I started bleeding. I turned pale immediately and

started crying. But I AM READY! What about our baby? I knew nothing about the risk of miscarriage in the first trimester.

We went to get an ultrasound (it didn't show anything in my uterus), and HCG levels were going down throughout the week. More blood tests, more ultrasounds, and more "I am so sorry" looks from nurses. My HCG is at zero now, the miscarriage process is over. The support of our families and friends helped us go through this. That's how I found out how many of my friends experienced early miscarriages. I am lucky to have my loving husband and so much support from people who love us. We are happy.

—— OUR ADVICE

Nobody tells you how devastating it can be to experience a miscarriage, and also how common it is. One in four pregnancies end in miscarriage and most happen in the first 12 weeks. It's so strange how one moment you can be pregnant and the next moment not. And life just goes on around you and to everyone else you appear the same as before. It's sad and confusing and no less so just because it was unplanned or you only just found out.

There are no hard and fast rules to how you might or should feel when you lose a baby. For some women it is life changing, for others it's an inconvenience and for many it's a sad episode that fades as time passes. However you feel, it's fine to feel that way and hopefully you have the support around you that you need.

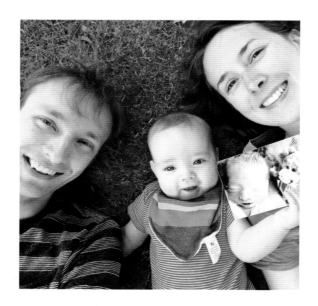

About pregnancy after loss

Georgia Keogh-Horgan @_abcdefgeorg
heyworlditshenry.com

Pregnancy after loss requires strength, in my case a strength born when my firstborn son Henry unexpectedly died. Strength to manage conflicting emotions; joy for this second child alongside grief for my first. The strength to hold on to hope while feeling so very afraid. It requires courage. To dare to try again. To let myself love another baby when I already love one who could not stay. To face a society uncomfortable with child loss, one quick to celebrate this new baby but unable to speak my missing child's name.

Pregnancy after loss is not a normal pregnancy. It is wanting the impossible, for both my children to be here. It is acknowledging the uncomfortable truth that had my first child lived, my second probably would not exist. It is wondering whether I could possibly love another child as much as I love my first, and feeling guilty for even thinking it.

Pregnancy after loss is never going to be easy but holding on to the knowledge that I had survived more than I ever thought possible, and that just like their brother this child would be worth it, I did it. And she is.

—— OUR ADVICE

To lose a baby at any stage of pregnancy or after the birth is devastating, and making the decision to have another baby is a very big deal. Pregnancy after a loss like this can be very difficult for women and their partners. It is a time that will probably be dominated by feelings of anxiety and fear. This is completely understandable.

There are things that you can do to try and help you through this tough time – talk to others who have been through the same thing. Talk to your midwife or doctor about your worries, and don't feel embarrassed to ask for extra scans or extra support if you feel you need it. No one will think you are wasting their time.

Don't feel pressured to buy lots of things or to get stuff ready for your baby. Take care of yourself. Take time to relax and eat well. However you feel is ok.

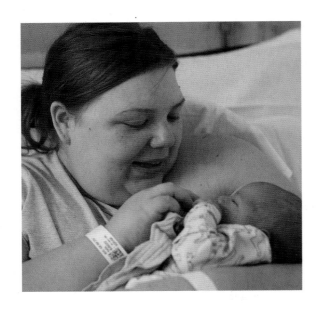

Plus-size motherhood doesn't have to be harder

Hollie Burgess @HolliePlus
Prettybigbutterflies.com

There are so many negative connotations surrounding being plus size and pregnant that I assumed it would be a long, hellish or even impossible journey for me. While I'm fully aware that all pregnancies and women are different, my plus-size pregnancies were amazing.

I conceived almost instantly and I had two really healthy and enjoyable pregnancies. No gestational diabetes, great blood pressure and I didn't put on any extra weight. Even though I was classified as morbidly obese on the BMI scale, pregnancy really agreed with my body and I had textbook pregnancies. I was classified as high risk, which was scary, but I understood that the professionals had their reasons. Extra measures were put in place, such as extra scans and blood-thinning injections, and my birthing options were limited. But the key for me was not to let it make me feel like a bad mum. This isn't about glorifying obesity. I'm just a plus-size mum, who had great pregnancies, healthy babies and really good experiences with healthcare professionals . . . and I'd do it all over again if I could get some more sleep.

—— OUR ADVICE

If you are obese, it is perfectly possible to conceive easily, have a perfect pregnancy and a textbook birth. It just may be a bit more worrying for you, and it might mean that you will need extra monitoring and perhaps some restrictions on your birth choices.

There are health risks associated with being obese when you are pregnant, which can't be ignored. It puts you and your baby at higher risk of complications such as miscarriage, gestational diabetes, high blood pressure and more. The probability is higher that you will have a bigger baby, which can make delivery more complicated. Obese women are more likely to need an instrumental delivery or an emergency caesarean section. The likelihood of having a stillbirth doubles if you have a BMI of over 30.

If you are overweight and considering starting a family, it is a good idea to try and lose some weight before you get pregnant. If you are overweight and already pregnant, though, please do not start trying to lose weight now. It's best to talk to your midwife or doctor about your diet. And remember, most women who are overweight will have a problem-free pregnancy and have a healthy baby – this is an important message to take away!

And obviously, being overweight does not stop you from being a brilliant parent, so do not let anyone suggest otherwise!

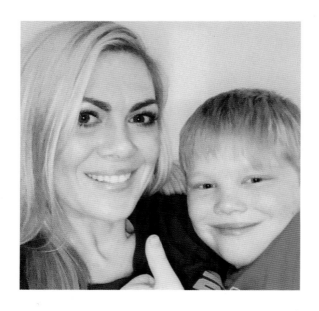

Ectopic pregnancy can be life-threatening

Bianca Carr @biancajaynecarr

I had the most intense, sharp pain ripping through my lower abdomen and tearing my insides. I went dizzy and was seeing stars. My hearing went muffled. Ten long seconds. Then it was gone.

That night I was kept awake by terrible period-like pain. The pain got worse and I woke up on the floor in the toilet, dripping in sweat and crippled with pain.

I was taken to hospital and was drifting in and out of consciousness and remember being raced down the corridor on a bed. Operating table next and then finally I woke up to a bag of blood hanging beside me, a drain out of my stomach and a very fetching wee bag.

I had been 7 weeks pregnant and the baby had grown in my fallopian tube. It had ruptured and I was bleeding internally. I needed life-saving surgery to remove my left tube and stop the bleeding. Three blood transfusions, a quick restart of the old ticker and I'm alive and kicking. I now only have one tube but I have had two awesome little boys since!

—— OUR ADVICE

An ectopic pregnancy is when a fertilised egg starts to grow in your fallopian tube rather than your womb. Sadly it is never possible to save the pregnancy and it is usually removed via surgery or by taking medication. In the UK around one in 90 pregnancies is ectopic.

Sometimes there are no symptoms at all and the ectopic pregnancy is not diagnosed until you have a scan.

SYMPTOMS CAN INCLUDE:
- irregular bleeding or brown/watery discharge
- tummy pains, sometimes on one side
- a missed period or pregnancy symptoms
- pain in the tip of your shoulder
- discomfort in your bottom when going to the loo

Sometimes the ectopic pregnancy can cause the tube to rupture which can then lead to internal bleeding. This is life-threatening and you should call an ambulance if your pain is sudden or severe or you start to feel lightheaded, dizzy, or you have fainted.

Most women who have had an ectopic pregnancy will be able to get pregnant again and luckily for most women, it is a one-off event.

—— CONTENTS

Your pregnancy

Whether your journey to this point was short or long, filled with joy or tinged with sadness, whether you're surprised to be here or you dreamt of this moment all your life, it doesn't matter. Pregnancy is an exciting yet nerve-wracking time of your life. You deserve excellent care and support and information from sources you can trust.

This chapter is full of stories and advice on the most common concerns of pregnancy and all the things that Nobody Tells You . . .

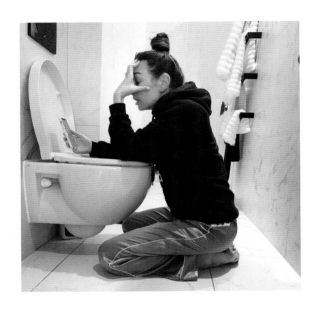

"Morning sickness" can last all day

Michelle Kennedy @peanut

We're super excited to have another little peanut on the way, and we feel so blessed. BUT, it wouldn't be fair of me to post a glowing picture without being completely honest about the realities of the first trimester.

The truth is, this has been a very rough 3+ months. I've been more sick than I thought possible and it's impacted every area of my life. Spending time lying on the tiles of your office bathroom trying to engage your brain, trying to excite your team about the quarter ahead while trying to swallow down some dry crackers, then at home trying to build Lego and interrupting it to run and kneel at the porcelain bowl has been overwhelming, exhausting and humbling, and I say that as someone who is building a company for mothers. I can't imagine what that is like for women in other sectors. You're at your most vulnerable, unable to share your news, desperate to keep this little life safe, and yet determined to keep everything going: home, work, life.

I've made loads of mistakes, I've been grumpy AF, I've been late to meetings getting out of the cab to vomit at the side of the road.

For all the women still going through it, or still on their journey to get there, I see you. We see you. You might not be at par, but you're doing great.

—— OUR ADVICE

"Morning Sickness" is an inaccurate description for many women. The nausea can last all day, or even arrive in the afternoon. It can be worse when you are hungry or tired or can be triggered by certain smells or motion. While some women compare the feeling to an all-day hangover, others actually vomit on a daily basis. Either way it can be an unpleasant start to what most hope will be a wonderful time in their lives.

On a positive note, feeling sick can be a sign that your pregnancy hormones are high, which is good for the growing baby. Nausea during the first few weeks of pregnancy is associated with a lower than average risk of miscarriage and may be the body's way of stopping you from taking in "poisons". It often improves somewhere between 14 and 16 weeks, but for some women it does last a bit longer.

Things that can help morning sickness

Eat as soon as you wake up, or even while still in bed.

Nibble on crackers or biscuits often, even in the night, especially if you wake up hungry during the night. Hunger can make the nausea worse. Keep a cracker, biscuit or banana on your bedside table!

Ginger in any form: fresh, tea, biscuits or sweets.

Acupressure bands (sea sickness bands) – these can be found in most chemists or online.

Rest as much as you can as tiredness can make it worse.

If it is affecting your work then it could be a good idea to tell your boss even if you are less than 12 weeks pregnant.

If you are being sick on the way to work or while out and about then take a plastic bag, bottle of water and chewing gum/toothbrush in your handbag.

If you cannot keep fluids down, you are losing weight and the sickness is affecting your day-to-day life you could be suffering from hyperemesis gravidarum.

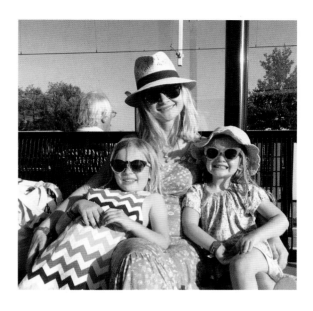

Hyperemesis gravidarum can affect you mentally and physically

Mandie Gower @mandiegower15

Puking multiple times an hour for twelve hours straight isn't normal. Most people just call it "really bad morning sickness", which is a bit like calling the Plague a touch of flu.

Mine started at 7 weeks with both pregnancies. At first, I felt I was a bit of a weakling so I soldiered on, puking my guts up from the moment I woke and discreetly vomiting on the Tube into carrier bags.

I lost 5kg, couldn't eat, and could barely hold down water. I tried three types of anti-sickness medication. Eventually, exhausted and delirious, I was hospitalised for the first time, but only after slumping on the floor of A&E for four hours, as sitting upright was intolerable. It took seven goes to insert the cannula as my veins had collapsed from dehydration but even then I felt like a fraud. 'Well, baby is very healthy!' chirped the doctor, as if wanting to feel the same was the height of selfishness.

Nobody tells you how depressing it is when you're discharged, knowing you'll be back. How guilty you feel for moaning when others so desperately want a baby. And how you'll understand why some women with HG choose to terminate their pregnancy. People just tell you to eat bloody ginger biscuits.

Instead they should tell you that you're a warrior just for getting out of bed. That complaining doesn't make you ungrateful. And that once your baby is born, it really is like a switch flicking. The curse is broken. You made it.

——— OUR ADVICE

Hyperemesis gravidarum is different from ordinary morning sickness or pregnancy-related nausea. It is characterised by excessive vomiting and often dehydration or loss of more than 5% of your pre-pregnancy weight.

If you are suffering from hyperemesis gravidarum it is not likely that any nausea remedies like ginger or sea sickness bands will offer much help. You may have trouble keeping anything down, even water, and in some instances you may require a stint in hospital on a drip to help rehydrate you.

If you cannot keep fluids down, or your sickness is affecting your day-to-day life, then please speak to your midwife or doctor as there are forms of medication that you can take to help with this that are safe for pregnant women and their babies.

Rest as much as you can, avoid smells, sounds and sights that may trigger your nausea. Find some emotional or psychological help if you need it. Sometimes just chatting things through with someone who has been through the same thing can help.

The UK charity Pregnancy Sickness Support (@pregnancysicknesssupport) is a lifeline to sufferers and their carers. They provide information on safe medical treatment options and run a peer support network which can be invaluable to women who are suffering from this debilitating condition.

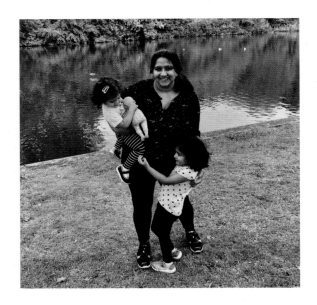

Being pregnant a second (or third) time isn't necessarily easier

Rohini Regunathan @claphammums
claphammums.com

The first time I was pregnant, I was a wreck. The second time around, I felt relaxed – your body should know the drill, right? I wasn't worried, and I started planning ahead, but I miscarried at 11 weeks.

Third time lucky, and with my third pregnancy, everything seemed ok – until 11 weeks, when I suddenly had heavy bleeding again. It felt like déjà vu and I was bracing for the heartbreak. The scan showed a threatened miscarriage, which meant taking it easy and holding my breath till the next scan. My anxiety was sky-high; every twitch made me wonder if I was miscarrying. But it was all fine!

In my third trimester, I developed calf pain and bouts of breathlessness. My GP was worried about blood clots. After a few rounds of Heparin injections and many scans, it turned out to be a scare.

I had assumed that my second time would be easier than my first, and I wasn't prepared for so much anxiety – it was exhausting. But after all the scares, the birth was anti-climactic; three pushes and she was here. And holding her, I forgot (most of) the stress!

—— OUR ADVICE

No two pregnancies are the same. You will meet some women who sail through the nine months without a bother. No sickness, no aches or pains, no scares, no anxiety, no stretch marks . . . they even have that fabled pregnancy 'glow'. Avoid these people at all costs – they are way too irritating to be around! (Just kidding.)

You may have it the other way around. Nausea, vomiting, pains, bleeding. Worrying that you are going to have a miscarriage. Heartburn, haemorrhoids, feeling heavy and short of breath. Extra hospital appointments for things that make you high risk, like family history, your age and sometimes your race. It is sometimes beyond your control and often very worrying.

Most women have an experience in between these two extremes. So do not fret if you feel you are off to a bad start. Most of these issues resolve themselves as the pregnancy progresses, and the rest as soon as your baby is born.

If you are ever worried about yourself or your baby and have any worrying symptoms, please do speak to your midwife or GP as soon as you can. Do not just sit at home googling things and making yourself more worried. For advice on bleeding, see pages 52–3.

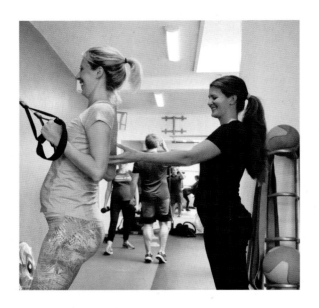

You can exercise during pregnancy

Heidi Skudder @theparentandbabycoach
theparentandbabycoach.com

Nobody tells you that you can stay fit and still carry out an exercise programme while pregnant. It was a revelation for me! Apparently keeping fit is actually now the way forward in helping towards a healthy baby and birth.

After spending the first trimester feeling constantly sick, I was desperate at 14 weeks to get back into my usual fitness regime. But everything I googled told me to be careful, that I had to take it easy and on some websites I read that it wasn't recommended. I felt like

I'd never get "myself" back and I was only a third of the way into pregnancy!

Finally at 20 weeks I found a trainer who introduced me to a whole new world of fitness during pregnancy. Their classes were tailored to the pregnant body – you can even do abs exercises if they are done safely and in the right way.

There needs to be more information on exercise in pregnancy, as the norm seems to still be to put your feet up and take it easy. So many women are scared of harming their baby when actually, it has far more benefits when done in the right way with the right support and advice.

—— OUR ADVICE

Vigorous exercise during pregnancy used to be seen as dangerous to the baby. But with no evidence to support this, doctors are increasingly encouraging pregnant women to get moving.

There are so many benefits to staying fit during your pregnancy. Evidence shows us that if you're fit you will reduce the likelihood of complications in late pregnancy and labour. Most importantly, being fit increases the likelihood of a "normal" vaginal birth and reduces the need for emergency C-section and assisted delivery. Giving birth is a physically demanding process, and often, the fitter you can be in preparation for this, the better!

Be careful, though: during pregnancy your body will produce increased amounts of a hormone called relaxin, which is designed to loosen your joints and muscles in preparation for the impending birth. This means that your joints are not as strong as usual and your balance may even be thrown off-kilter, so it is important to bear this in mind when considering doing any exercise.

Swimming, walking, yoga and pilates are great forms of exercise that are gentle on your joints. Steer clear of vigorous sports . . . no ice hockey or tae kwon do! Trained athletes can often keep going with their chosen sport until quite late in pregnancy.

If you are taking up a new sport, please chat to your doctor or midwife about this. Listen to your body. If you feel out of breath, feel any pain or have any bleeding when you're exercising you should stop immediately and speak to your midwife.

> There are leaflets that describe these exercises in confusing detail, but I always just used to tell patients, "Imagine you're sitting in a bath full of eels and you don't want any of them getting in."
>
> Adam Kay
> *This Is Going to Hurt*

How to do pelvic floor exercises

Genevieve Westoby-Lloyd @genevievewestoby

The only real advice I received about pelvic floor exercises before having my baby was medical professionals asking, "You are doing your pelvic floors, aren't you?" and that was it. No discussion of technique, frequency . . . nothing.

They weren't given any kind of importance, seemingly an after-thought as you were leaving your class or midwife appointment. That's how antenatal education and check-ups seemed to me – they focused on the big event – B-Day! How you were going to get through the birth, not how you were going to get through THE

REST OF YOUR LIFE having pushed an actual human being out. Unless like me your baby ended up exiting through the sunroof . . .

"Sorted" I thought! No perineal damage for me, no unnecessary stretching of my foof, and my pelvic floor should be more taut than the drumskin of a Glastonbury headliner. Not so, apparently! The act of carrying a baby itself puts a lot of strain on the pelvic floor. I was not prepared for the first-time feeling of pissing myself when I needed a wee and sneezed!

———— OUR ADVICE

It is never too late to start doing your pelvic floor exercises. Ideally you should start your pelvic floor exercises before you even get pregnant, and if not then you should start them during your pregnancy, but if you didn't manage that, then don't worry, you can start now! Even if you're 39 weeks pregnant, two days or ten years postnatal, it is never too late to start squeezing!

You use your pelvic floor muscles for weeing, pooing and having sex and you need these muscles to be strong if you don't want to pee yourself every time you sneeze, cough, laugh, run or jump.

It can make you feel a bit funny inside or shaky the first few times you do them, but it's similar to when you start to work any muscle properly for the first time (like when you try to plank or do sit-ups for the first time). But if you persevere they become easy and natural and part of your daily life and you will be so thankful for them the first time you have to get on a bouncy castle with your child!

So how do you do pelvic floor exercises?

Most women have a vague idea that exercising the pelvic floor is important, but many are not sure why. And even more are not sure how.

WHAT IS THE PELVIC FLOOR?

The pelvic floor is a set of muscles that are positioned between the pubic bone (at the front – inside your pubes) and your tailbone (the bottom of your spine, just above your bum crack!). The muscles sit like a hammock and hold all your pelvic organs in place. This includes your bladder, bowel, uterus and vagina.

WHY IS IT IMPORTANT?

When these muscles are working well they support the bladder and bowel and work with them to let you pee and poo when you need to. They also support your vagina and are important for your sex life (being able to clench and make it tighter rather than loose). If they are not working well then you may experience urinary incontinence (wee), faecal incontinence (poo) or flatus incontinence (fart), none of which are pleasant!

—— HOW DOES PREGNANCY AFFECT THE PELVIC FLOOR?

As you can imagine, the weight of a growing baby in your uterus is going to put stress on this muscle and regardless of whether or not you push a baby out of your vagina or have a caesarean section, the pelvic floor will feel different after you have had a baby. The muscles will be weakened, which can put you at risk of several nasty things such as:

- Incontinence (weeing, pooing and farting)
- Prolapse (where your pelvic organs drop down and sometimes fall out towards the opening of your vagina)
- Reduced sexual sensitivity (which you may not care about so much in the first few weeks after giving birth . . . but you will do again one day)

—— HOW CAN I STRENGTHEN MY PELVIC FLOOR?

Regular pelvic floor exercises, sometimes called Kegels, can help strengthen the pelvic floor. Just like any muscle in your body, regular training and use will keep it in good condition.

—— HOW TO DO PELVIC FLOOR EXERCISES

Pelvic floor guru Jane Wake @janewakeuk gives this advice:
"To find your pelvic floor muscles, imagine you are stopping a wee and pull up the muscles in your vagina. Then, imagine you want to stop a fart and contract the muscles in your back passage and pull them up too. Try and hold these muscles up at the same time and imagine them coming to meet in your centre. And now release them. It is important to be able to release the muscles after you have contracted them."

AIM TO TRY AND DO THE FOLLOWING
EXERCISES 10 TIMES EACH, 5 TIMES A DAY:

We know it's a lot but you will thank us for it in the long run!

- Stop a fart, then stop a wee, pulling up gradually and then releasing slowly
- Stop a fart, then stop a wee and imagine your pelvic floor is a lift going up through five floors. Pull up to the first floor, then the second, then the third, fourth and fifth! Release and let the lift go all the way back down again (slowly if you can)
- Stop a fart, stop a wee, pull up and then release in quick succession

The NHS 'Squeezy' app is great for reminding you to do your pelvic floor exercises.

You can also get specialised equipment which is designed to improve your technique and can record the strength of your pelvic floor.

If you are having any trouble with your pelvic floor, either before, during or after pregnancy, please go and see your GP or a women's health physio.

Good luck, and remember – it's never too late to start!

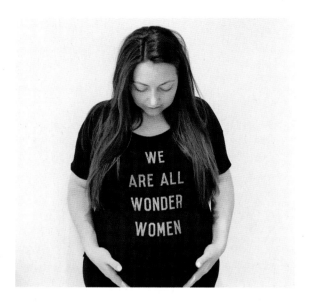

Strangers seem to think it's ok to touch your bump

Charlotte Archibald @charl_archie_

Why do people feel they have free rein to touch your bump or pass comment on it? I've been told, by people I have never met before:

"Ooh you carry large, don't you?"

"Wow that's a massive bump for 7 months!"

"Are you sure it's not twins?"

"My daughter-in-law is 35 weeks pregnant and her bump is half the size of yours!"

And my personal favourite: "Are you drinking too much water?"

There's something mystic and compelling about a pregnancy

bump that makes perfect strangers feel like they have carte blanche to make deeply personal comments and assertions about your ability to grow a baby. Is it because your bump is so visible, so obviously not a normal part of you, that people think it is somehow fair game for anyone to comment on or touch? Like a jaunty hat or a sale tag accidentally left hanging out the back of a jacket?

I personally love how huge my stomach is – I love the constant reminder that my new little human is growing nicely inside me and is on its way soon. Before I know it, the baby will be out in the big world and I know I'll miss my "mahoosive belly" when it's (almost) gone.

—— OUR ADVICE

Yes, it's true. People get excited when they see a pregnant woman and feel the need to touch, pass comment or give you some form of advice which may or may not be helpful. Brace yourself for when the baby arrives, as this sort of unsolicited attention can be even more prevalent once you are pushing a newborn around!

Many women find it easiest to simply smile, nod politely and say "thank you" (possibly through gritted teeth). Every once in a while, there is likely to be a snippet of something useful, so hold out for those precious moments!

If you really can't stand to be touched then please don't feel embarrassed to push away a stray hand and maybe just explain that your skin is very sensitive.

Everyone carries their baby differently and it is not a good idea to compare your bump with others, or listen to the comments of people without medical training as it does not really mean anything. If you feel worried about the size of your bump then please do speak to your midwife about this as he or she will be able to reassure you.

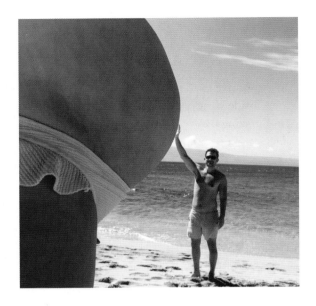

Your bump is amazing

Lexie Allman @lexsentials
lexsentials.com

Nobody tells you to embrace your pregnant body! I have never loved my body so much as during my pregnancy. As my bump grew, so did the pride and joy I felt. I felt so lucky to be able to carry it around with me everywhere I went, knowing that we were doing everything together. And on my babymoon, I very proudly wore bikinis, showing off the body that we had together become as one.

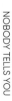

Even if you have never loved your body, you can't help but look at your bump in awe in that last trimester. It's an absolute miracle to be able to grow an actual real-life human being (or multiple human beings) inside your tummy, so please stop for a second and celebrate this amazing fact and think about documenting it for the future! It's awesome to take some photos to be able to show your children where they grew and it's mind-blowing to look back and see the changes your body has gone through.

You can take a shot of yourself every week and make a cool montage of your growing bump. You can do the Demi Moore-style naked shot. You can do secret selfies in the mirror. You can share them or you can hide them away. It doesn't matter, just be proud and take a snap, you won't regret it!

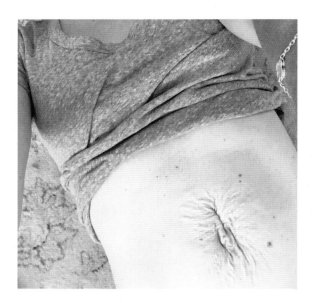

Stretch marks
aren't so bad

Saskia Boujo @factsoflife.ed
saskiaboujo.com

My tummy has a hundred stories to tell and this is what it looks
like after two laparoscopies, one hysteroscopy to have my tubes
removed, four rounds of IVF, and three C-sections to get my three
breech girls out. Despite all my efforts with coconut, almond, cocoa
butter and rose oil, I am left with these loose flappy bits of skin and
stretch marks (that weirdly glow in the dark), a horrific raised and
bumpy keloid C-section scar, and my belly button lost somewhere in
the middle of it all!

But . . . I wouldn't change it for the world. Look at what I've made – three babies. Now, I make sure I am naked as much as possible, letting it all hang out to show them I am (kinda) ok with it. I accept that there are those that get their iron-flat tummies back in a few weeks with not a mark in sight, and that there is me who is learning to embrace a one-piece swimsuit!

I've never been brave enough to show it to anyone but my husband, my mum and my sister and my girls. Now I'll show you. And cry a bit. Who knows, maybe I'll rock a bikini again some day for the world to see.

—— OUR ADVICE

Whether or not you get stretch marks during your pregnancy will depend mostly upon your genetics. If your mother or sister had stretch marks during their pregnancies, the chances are that you will too. No amount of lotions or potions will keep these marks at bay, so please do not be fooled into spending a fortune on creams that promise the earth.

Some women swear by special oils, but while these can help with the discomfort of your skin stretching and keep your skin moisturised and in some cases even help fade stretch marks after the birth, they will not stop them from appearing.

Your stretch marks are just a reminder of what your body has achieved, so try and love them if you can as they are there to stay!

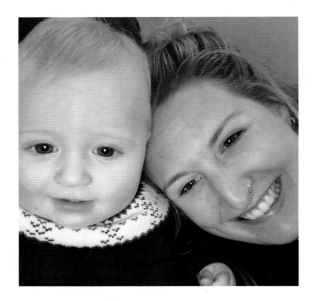

You might not feel so happy

Juliet Rood @julietpickle

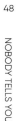

Sometimes being pregnant doesn't fill you with joy and excitement. My pregnancy was sadly riddled with anxiety and utter fear of the unknown. I wanted a family but fell pregnant very quickly and it was a shock. I hated pregnancy; I felt huge and miserable – I had very few other pregnancy symptoms but I felt totally out of control and as a very organised person I felt I couldn't cope. I couldn't sleep and was constantly worried about my pregnancy, the birth and impending motherhood. I felt really panicked about the huge changes ahead. All I could think about was how much my life was going to change for the worse; how it would affect my relationship, how I would no longer have a social life and how much responsibility I would have once the baby was born.

I desperately wanted to join in with my husband's excitement but I couldn't and I felt like I was letting him down. I spoke to my midwife and straight away she arranged some extra support, which was great and really helped.

Now my son is here and it is amazing. I can't wait to expand our family in the future but mostly I look forward to hopefully enjoying the next pregnancy now that I know the happy ending.

—— OUR ADVICE

Traditionally most attention has been directed towards psychological problems after the pregnancy. But we now suspect that at least one in ten women may have psychological problems such as anxiety, depression or panic attacks during pregnancy. Around 50% of pregnancies are unplanned and women are sometimes unsupported and have no extended family network. They may find themselves isolated and far away from friends and family or may have previous history of psychological problems. And sometimes there may be no obvious reasons to explain why you are feeling this way.

Fortunately these problems do not affect the growth or development of the baby and do not seem to change the way that the body works in late pregnancy or labour. However, if you do have psychological problems it may make pregnancy seem a lot longer and more difficult than it otherwise would be. The side effects, discomfort, aches and pains may be more difficult to tolerate.

If you feel that you may be suffering from any psychological problems while you are pregnant then please speak to your midwife or doctor who will advise you on the best course of action to take.

How can I explain what's all in my head
It feels like I'm tangled up in a web
A path unknown laid out before me
Paralysed with fear, when two become three

We are told of joy and happiness galore
But how do we know what really lies in store
I've not felt excitement like everyone said
Instead I am terrified of what lies ahead

I'm scared of the birth and being in pain
I know that our life will never be the same
What if he loves me a little less?
What if I can't do it and I'm a total mess

It feels like friends are already drifting
I know for sure that priorities are shifting
It's hard to explain what this baby has cost
I feel like my identity is already lost

Riddled with guilt for not feeling happy inside
I'm surely not ready for this incredible ride
I hope that when the baby comes out
A gush of love will at long last sprout

As the due date draws closer day by day
A seed of excitement is hinting display
Reality has hit, I'm no longer number one
It's a bit of a shock, becoming a mum

Juliet Rood @julietpickle

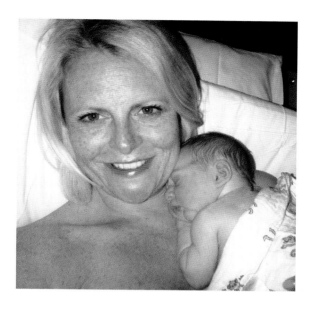

Bleeding in early pregnancy can be so worrying

Becca Maberly @amotherplace
amotherplace.com

Five days before my 12-week scan I felt a trickle between my legs. Blood was dripping out of me at an alarming rate. I sat on the loo and more flowed out until there was a plop and something dropped out of me into the loo. There was no pain or discomfort – just the feeling of complete shock as the thing I presumed was my baby just dropped into the loo. I couldn't bring myself to look at it again.

I drove myself to the Early Pregnancy Assessment Unit, assuming that a scan would just confirm the bad news I expected. But no, my baby was flipping and moving around inside me. The sense of relief was incredible. My baby was still alive! The sonographer could not see any reason for the bleeding. My cervix was closed and my placenta was in a good position away from my cervix.

She explained that it could have been scar tissue that had been building up since implantation, and while most women absorb this back into their bodies, sometimes this does not happen and the womb will expel it. It was so frightening but my son arrived happy and healthy six months later!

—— OUR ADVICE

BLEEDING IN EARLY PREGNANCY

Bleeding in early pregnancy is common and happens in at least one in four pregnancies. It does not mean you have lost the baby. You do need a scan and this can usually be arranged by your GP or you can head straight to your Early Pregnancy Unit (EPU) where you can be seen at short notice and hopefully reassured. In an emergency you can go to your local Accident and Emergency Department. Most hospitals have emergency gynaecology services so can arrange scans even at weekends.

It is always alarming but often your pregnancy will continue normally, ending with a healthy mother and baby.

Bleeding in early pregnancy can occur for a variety of reasons. Most of the time the bleeding is coming from inside the uterus but occasionally it can be due to problems on the cervix or elsewhere in the genital tract.

Sometimes at approximately 10–14 days after conception there can be a small amount of blood which coincides with the embryo embedding in the wall of the uterus. This is called an implantation bleed. This diagnosis can only be made in retrospect after a scan confirms the pregnancy is alive and well.

Bleeding in pregnancy can sometimes be an early warning of a miscarriage, especially if you have cramping or period-type pains. An early scan performed through the vagina can usually reveal if the pregnancy is going well or not.

Most commonly, early pregnancy problems are dealt with urgently in a designated Early Pregnancy Unit which will be staffed by skilled nurses, doctors and sonographers.

Occasionally, however, the scans are inconclusive and need to be repeated, sometimes with serial blood tests to measure levels of the pregnancy hormone HCG.

BLEEDING IN LATER PREGNANCY

Any bleeding later in your pregnancy requires immediate attention at a hospital where your midwife or doctor will listen to your story, examine you, listen to the baby's heartbeat, and arrange a scan and blood tests.

Occasionally women experience bleeding from the neck of the womb, which is not so serious but still needs careful examination and assessment. At some stage your cervix may need to be inspected (using a speculum, like during a smear test). Most of the time the bleeding is mild and settles quickly. The blood is usually maternal (your blood) not fetal (your baby's) so will not affect the growth or development of the baby.

However, recurrent bleeding can sometimes interfere with the function of the placenta and this can affect the growth of the baby. You may need extra monitoring and sometimes early delivery of your baby may be advised.

—— CONTENTS

Your birth

Thinking about giving birth for the first time can feel daunting. It is important that there are no nasty surprises in store, so it's good to know about all your options and the risks and benefits associated with each one. Birth does not have to be scary, it can be positive and beautiful, but you have to keep an open mind and maintain realistic expectations.

This chapter explores the many different ways of giving birth and is full of momentous and affirmative things that Nobody Tells You . . .

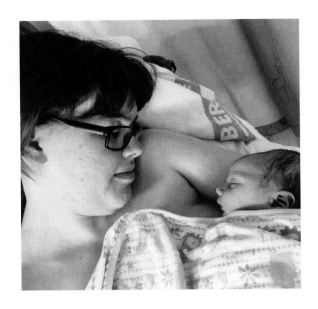

Birth plans do not always go according to plan

Lydia Banfield @lydirose16

Writing my birth plan was really exciting, I felt able to think and consider what I would really like for my birth. We had talked at our antenatal classes about different types of birth, pain relief etc. I decided I only wanted gas and air, a water birth and DEFINITELY not to be stuck to a bed, no epidural or C-section.

What I didn't plan for was for my birth plan not to go to plan! My beautifully printed and typed birth plan didn't even come out of my hospital bag! I was stuck on a bed for hours, having an epidural, and ended up with an emergency C-section.

It's great to be prepared and consider what you would and wouldn't like but sometimes that doesn't account for the unplanned and unexpected nature of birth. I really struggled following my birth as it wasn't the picture-perfect birth we were sold at our classes or what I had imagined for myself, and honestly I felt I had let everyone down and felt so guilty. Fortunately my health visitor recognised that I was struggling. I was referred to a fantastic psychologist from the perinatal mental health team who diagnosed me with PTSD and supported me in combating these flashbacks and feelings of guilt that my birth plan hadn't gone to plan.

—— OUR ADVICE

Investing time in writing lengthy, rigid and detailed birth plans can sometimes contribute to a sense of failure or sadness if things do not go according to this plan. Feeling like you have "failed" at giving birth is tragic and unfair. No one should feel that they failed at something over which they didn't even have full control.

Maybe we can encourage women to express their "birth wishes" instead of writing a birth plan. Perhaps if we just renamed this document, and asked women to jot down some things they feel passionate about or worried about, then we would take the emphasis off the "planning" aspect and free up our expectations. This could help reduce the likelihood of feeling let down in the all-important postnatal period.

If we make sure that women and their partners understand the physiology of labour, what happens when Mother Nature doesn't get it quite right, and what their options are, then we can help them to form more realistic expectations. Let's encourage them to express these expectations, hopes and fears but not get too bogged down with the details.

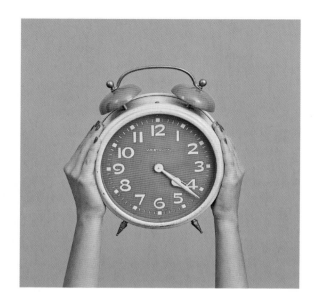

About early labour

Beccy Hands @beccy_hands
beccyhands.co.uk

Nobody told me that it could go on for DAYS – literally! I had a back-to-back baby, and the longest latent phase known to man. I was so ready for my active home birth and to finally meet a baby that kept me waiting for two weeks postdate, that I peaked too soon. I was up, bouncing on my ball, crab-walking up and down the stairs and counting every contraction WAY too early! I'd worn myself out before labour had even started (and I should have known better – I am a doula and I work with women in labour).

I wish somebody had reminded me to ignore those first twinges – to go to bed and sleep or rest until I couldn't rest any more. I wish someone had recalled that active labour comes later, when you are actually in established labour and that focusing on the contractions too soon is literally like watching paint dry!

Finally, I wish somebody had told me that a long latent phase isn't always a bad thing, and that with rest, support and a whole load of digging deep for patience – you can still end up with a wonderful delivery and a really positive birth experience.

—— OUR ADVICE

Early labour is also known as the latent phase of labour, and the big variable in labour is the length of this latent phase. This is often determined by the position of the baby rather than the size. In some cases, the latent phase can go on for a day or two. For most women this will be very manageable, and in some cases you may not even know you are in latent labour – you may just feel more frequent and stronger Braxton Hicks (tightenings) than normal.

About 20% of women may have a painful and extended labour because of the position of the baby – the most common of which is called occipito-posterior (OP) which is also known as "back to back". This means the baby is positioned on its back with its head facing skyward rather than facing down in the ideal position. OP can be diagnosed by a careful examination of the tummy or a scan, or when in labour, by an internal examination. A long early labour can really demoralise and discourage many women because they do not realise or had not anticipated it taking so long or being in pain before active labour even begins.

What can you do in early labour?

If you are low risk and the midwife or doctor is not concerned about your condition, you may be advised to stay at home until you are in established labour. If you have gone into the hospital you may be advised to head home again, depending on any risk factors and how much pain you're in and how you're coping.

Try to sleep and eat if you can. If you can manage to nap or eat then it is likely that you are not yet in established labour. If you're hungry, a light meal is better than a three-course banquet, as your digestion will slow down as labour progresses and when active labour begins, your body will be keen to rid itself of excess food it's carrying! It will look for the quickest way to do this, and in some cases women find themselves vomiting during the active stage.

Oral painkillers such as paracetamol, hypnobirthing, or a TENS machine may help the pain. Walking around can help and is a good form of distraction and it's thought that keeping upright and mobile can help labour to progress.

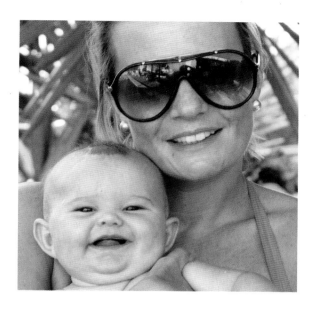

Contractions hurt!

Claire Dew @claireldew

Nobody can prepare you for what contractions are really like. Some people say that nobody told them how painful contractions are and it felt like a shock when they started to get painful. Well I totally believe in being honest and telling people how it actually feels.

Before I gave birth I had the worst pre-birth fear possible and I cried every time I thought about the fast-approaching due date; I couldn't watch anything related to childbirth as I was so petrified. But even though I was crippled with fear I really felt like hearing about other people's real experiences (every different version!) absolutely helped me to prepare myself mentally for what was ahead.

Both of my births were the most intensely painful thing I have ever experienced, the second without any drugs or anything at all. But I can honestly say I was psychologically prepared because of other people's honesty and this helped me to be mentally stronger during my own labour.

Above all else both births were also completely worth every single second of the pain and I would do it all again in a heartbeat to get the amazing priceless treasure at the end!

—— OUR ADVICE

Yes, contractions are very painful for most women. We say this not to scare you, but to prepare you. It is really important that you are aware that they are painful so that when you feel the pain you are not shocked or frightened that something is going wrong. We have heard of women doing classes where they teach you that with the right mental attitude, it does not have to hurt. This is not true. It is possible to learn to control your reactions to pain, but you cannot make it vanish completely. Breathing rhythmically or practising hypnobirthing can really help you to do this.

Most women feel contractions in their tummy and describe them as being like very strong period pains that come and go while their tummy becomes rock hard. Some women feel contractions in their back and this can feel like very strong back pain that comes and goes.

If you are finding the pain unbearable then you have the option of pain relief. This is what epidurals were invented for! There should be no shame or sense of failure because you use pain relief while giving birth. You wouldn't have a tooth pulled out without pain relief, would you?

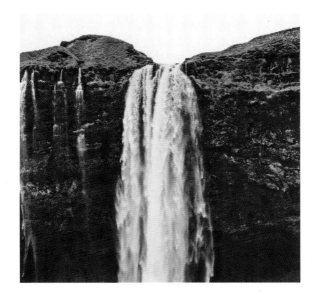

About the bodily fluids!

Hannah Rowlinson @hannahrowl

Nobody tells you that while you are in labour you might cover your partner in not one, not two but three kinds of bodily fluid! In labour, I did the longest wee of my life. I had to do it into a bedpan as they wanted to monitor my blood-sugar level. Mid-wee, I bellowed at my husband that the bedpan was filling and I couldn't stop and he had to move it and get me another!

I should mention here that I had already vomited on my husband. Anyway he bends down, as I'm still weeing away, he quickly grabs the bedpan with ONE HAND. The bedpan was full to the brim and the contents went EVERYWHERE! Covered my husband and the whole of the floor. He grabs multiple towels and starts mopping up.

I am still weeing.

A couple of seconds pass . . . Then there's a splash. More like a tsunami actually. My waters had just broken. My poor husband, who was still mopping up the contents of the bedpan incident just a few seconds earlier, was hit with yet another tidal wave of my bodily fluid.

Yeah. So. Nobody told me I would wee and puke on my husband and then GUSH all over him too!

——— OUR ADVICE

This is why it is a good idea for the partners to take a change of clothes to the hospital! Some women do vomit in labour. This is often because their digestive systems slow down while they are in labour and their guts may need to eject whatever is in there at the time. Sometimes you may vomit during the transition phase which is when labour is at its most painful and you are really exerting yourself.

It is also important to empty your bladder when you are in labour as you need an empty bladder to make room for the baby to descend through your pelvis!

As for your waters, you can't dictate how and when they will go! Some women have a small trickle and others have the big gush! Your birth partner doesn't need a plastic poncho like they're heading for Niagara Falls, but they might want to bring some spare clothes just in case!

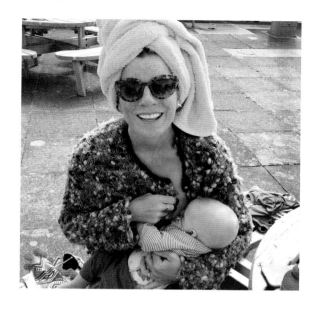

You might poo
during labour

Philippa Excell @phillyfitnesshenley

Nobody tells you that you might poo in front of your partner and that he might have to wipe your bum! My first daughter, Minnie, was born in a water bath at the hospital and it was all very relaxed and there was no poo which I was very proud of. Bessie, my second child, came really quickly in the waiting room as I walked in, so that was very dramatic but still no poo!

However, Dexter, my third child, also came very fast but luckily I had a room to myself. I remember pushing during a contraction and suddenly, I could smell something bad and realised it was me and I had done a poo on the floor! The midwife, for some reason, wasn't in the room so I was shouting at my hubby to clean the poo off the floor and wipe my bum before the nurse returned! That was the only thing I could focus on, so maybe that was a good distraction?! I have no idea where the poo went but I have an awful feeling that he just put it in the bin. I can't think about it without cringing and laughing at the same time!

——— OUR ADVICE

You won't always do a poo when you are giving birth, but if you do it's really not a big deal. The midwives and doctors have seen it all before and they will whisk it away with complete professionalism. You should also know that if you do push a poo out it's usually a good sign that you're pushing well and that the baby is close behind.

And while we are on the subject . . . you know how some people suggest you eat a hot curry to get things going and help induce labour? There is no evidence to show that this works and you should know that no one wants to see that vindaloo making its way out again the next day in the birthing pool or on the bed. Ok?

If you feel very nervous about doing a poo in labour and are worried that it may stop you pushing effectively then please speak to your midwife or doctor about using a glycerol suppository which can help you to empty your bowels before you are in active labour.

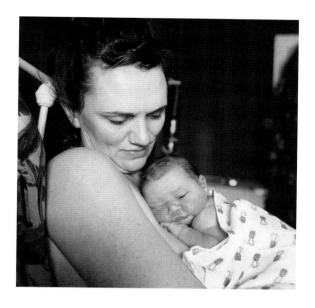

How to push

Victoria Emes @victoriaemes
victoriaemes.com

You've probably heard the analogy that pushing a baby out of your vadge is like squeezing an orange out of your nostril – and it's not far wrong. My second baby was yielding a head of such gigantic proportions that it felt more like an un-lubed bowling ball was smashing its way through my cervix. Thankfully she shot out so quickly that the sensation, although fucking intense, was literally over in a matter of minutes (17 to be precise).

    With my first labour the pushing stage was incredibly slow and drawn out. It took five long, knackering hours to convince that peanut to exit my womb and with every push he would move a few centimetres down before deciding "fuck this" and retracting right back up to where he'd come from. Although the descent for each of my labours was different, the actual moment of crowning felt exactly the same. The only way I can describe the act of your flaps stretching to betsy to accommodate a human skull is likening it to the sensation of a Chinese burn – but on your actual vagina. Ring of fire is one thing, but minge of fire is a whole other ball game. But honestly, if I could do it again tomorrow, I would. Giving birth to my children has been the most empowering experience of my life. I never realised just how strong and capable I am and it left me feeling like a fucking warrior. Women are amazing!

—— OUR ADVICE

If you have had no pain relief, when the time comes to push you will know! There is no alternative and you will know what to do. The nature of the contractions changes and normally most women will feel an intense pressure in their bottoms and the feeling of needing to push something out. Because of this sensation, for many women the pushing is automatic and instinctive, but you can optimise your technique with your midwife's support. Long pushes are better than short ones. Contractions last about 60 seconds, so it should be possible to do anything from two to five long pushes in that time.

The best way of pushing is with a lungful of air, mouth closed with chin on your chest, pushing downwards, using your lungful of air as a piston. Some women describe the pushing as like doing a massive poo. You should be aware that you might not progress with every contraction and every push. Sometimes the baby might move three steps forward two steps back, which can be discouraging if you are trying your hardest. But don't worry, this is normal.

—— WHAT IF YOU HAVE HAD AN EPIDURAL?

If you have had an epidural you will not get that same sensation of needing to push. You do not need to start pushing as soon as you are fully dilated – you may be able to wait for a while to allow the baby's head to come down and to let the epidural wear off a bit to increase sensation to allow you to feel the way to push.

If you decide to try and do this then you would be advised to lay off the top-ups of epidural. This is obviously something that will only happen if you want it to. If the pain is too much then you may have to have more epidural top-ups. If you cannot feel anything then the midwife will tell you when to push – she will know when your contractions are coming and will let you know and guide you with the pushing.

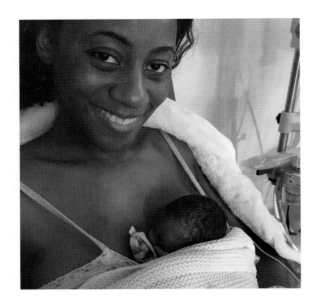

It might happen earlier than you expected

Charmaine White @twhinteriors
thewhitehouseinteriors.com

I woke at 4am with twinges, but being 29 weeks pregnant, I hadn't done antenatal classes or read any books yet, so I didn't know what was happening. I started bleeding so we went to the hospital. Everyone kept calm and no one told me I was in labour until I was hooked up to the monitor and they could see that my baby was ok.

As stressful as it might sound being told that your baby is on its way at 29 weeks, all the midwives and doctors were so calm that it made the whole experience relatively serene. Three hours and three pushes later my daughter was born. She only weighed 1360g, which I am told was a good weight for her gestation. It sounds tiny, but she didn't seem that small when I saw her because she was very long. When I was able to do skin-to-skin with her a few hours later, I put her on my chest and her legs stretched out all the way down my torso.

She was whisked off to NICU, where she remained for eight weeks in an incubator. I was there with her every day from 8am to 8pm, expressing litres of milk and giving her lots of skin-to-skin cuddles. I was obviously worried about her but I could see that she was getting the best care from the doctors and nurses on the neonatal ward, and I had great faith that she would be ok.

—— OUR ADVICE

Premature or preterm labour is defined as labour that starts before 37 weeks. In the UK, around eight out of 100 babies are born prematurely. If you're less than 37 weeks and experience any of the following symptoms, call your midwife/maternity unit immediately:

- Regular contractions or tightenings
- Pressure in your rectum or pelvic area
- Period-type pains in your tummy or back
- A show (this is when the mucus plug comes away from your cervix: gooey, bloody discharge)
- Bleeding
- Loss of fluid from your vagina (either a gush or a trickle)

If you are in labour, it may be possible to give you medication to slow things down or even stop them. You may also be given steroids to help mature your baby's lungs to get them ready for breathing if they are born early. Babies born before 37 weeks are often not yet fully developed, so they will often need some extra care from the neonatal unit. Latest statistics for the UK show that delivery at 31 weeks onwards has a 95% chance of survival, and from 34 weeks, the chances are similar to being at full term.

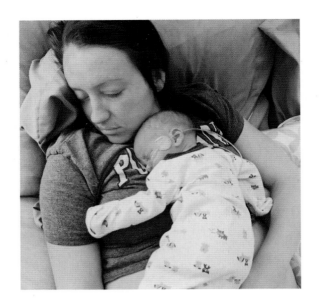

Things don't always go according to plan but it's ok

Cassandra Hall @cassiesuehall

Nobody tells you that your plans may all go out of the window but it will still be ok. My planned home birth turned into a hospital induction at 37 weeks but it was still a beautiful experience. It was a whirlwind. I had been fighting a sinus infection leading up to the induction and I was completely exhausted.

I had every intention to do this naturally but towards the end I was DONE. My midwife looked at me and said, "Cassie I need you to push." I replied back not so nicely . . . "And I need YOU to get me an epidural!" They kept telling me the baby would be here before the epidural. I didn't believe them and made them call for the anaesthetist. He was with another patient (btw, why do they only have ONE of those miracle workers in the whole hospital?!) Judea was born about five minutes later and I never got the epidural. I haemorrhaged and he was whisked away to the NICU (Neonatal Intensive Care Unit).

Things didn't go as planned but I still had such a beautiful experience. So many amazing things happened in the midst of all the pain and exhaustion. I wouldn't change it for the world.

—— OUR ADVICE

Your birth can be a positive experience even if it's not the one you imagined. There can often be too much emphasis on trying to plan for your birth. It's not like a room service menu – you can't tick the box asking for a painless birth with no stitches please! It's a real shame to hear about women who have just had babies who are sad, angry or sometimes totally confused because they did not get the birth they had planned and are asking "What happened? What did I do wrong?"

If your antenatal class, the book you read or the people you chat to do not give you an honest and realistic idea of how babies are born then they are doing you a disservice. You need to understand what happens when the textbook birth plans go out of the window, what your options are and what the risks associated with these options are.

If you are in a safe environment, surrounded by medical staff that you trust and supported by a confident birth partner, then even the most medicalised of births can feel special.

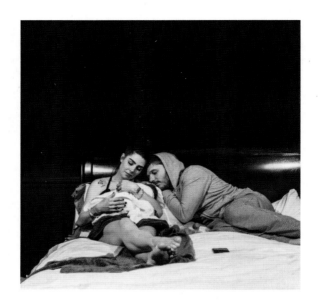

Birth can be perfect

Lucy Johnson-Reid @absolutely.fabulucy

I've had four very different births, I was a bit worried about having a home birth for my last birth but knew it was for me. I am a hypnobirthing lover and I also love a pool birth and my last two births were quite fast with no problems, so I was a "good candidate".

Ziggy was born in a pool at the end of our bed. The pool wasn't warm enough so they repeatedly filled two big Le Creuset bowls to get the right temperature for the birth. The children were in the room until about 15 minutes before he was born, they then went downstairs with Nanny and Grandad to have breakfast while Mummy completed the last slog.

I was totally silent, I was so calm, I took in every sound, feeling, twinge, I knew EXACTLY what my body was doing. I was in control, I was a warrior, I even managed to keep my shit together in the transition stage (which is the part where you go "right that's it, I can't do this, I'm going home"). The midwife didn't even know I had birthed Ziggy's head. I made sure I felt his head while he was head out and his body was still in – as this was my last baby I wanted to experience it all.

With the next push he was born, I caught him and I put him straight on my chest, nobody had touched us, it was like magic. The boys were in the room within about four minutes to meet their brother. I got into bed, delivered my placenta and literally didn't move all day, I lay in bed sniffing my new beautiful naked bambino, getting every bit of skin-to-skin love we could. I'm so happy that I got to experience that, it was the perfect end to my birthing days.

—— OUR ADVICE

Birth can be absolutely beautiful when it all goes according to plan. When Mother Nature does her thing right and you experience such a positive birth, it can feel very special indeed.

It is hard to try and manage your expectations about your birth as you often only hear about the extremes – the amazing birth or the horror story. And quite often it's all down to luck. We hope you enjoy this beautiful story and it doesn't make you feel sad if you didn't get your dream birth. It is just meant to inspire.

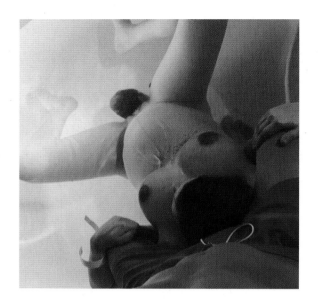

Water births can be amazing

Francesca De Paolis @frandepaolis

From when I was a child I always loved being in water, so when I was pregnant I really hoped for a water birth, though I knew it definitely wasn't a given. So I feel very lucky that both of my babies were born in water.

I was at 10cm when I arrived at the hospital and the midwife told me it was too late for a water birth. But I begged her and she ran the water for me, we dimmed the lights and put on our playlist. As soon as I got in the pool I felt a sensation of tranquility, the surges were less intense and I was more in control of what I was doing.

I held on to my husband's legs for support as I focused on getting my baby out calmly. My labour from start to finish was 12 hours but the active birth part was 1 hour and 12 minutes, all of which felt relatively calm. The water made me feel weightless and allowed me to move around easily to find my perfect birthing position.

I remember this moment so clearly when my daughter's head was poking out and it was a couple of minutes before the next surge. I asked the midwife if I could stroke her hair, which I did. I could see the side of her little face looking out into the water . . . her first glimpse of the world. Just magical. I asked my husband to get the camera to capture this precious moment. It feels so right that she is a little Pisces too.

—— OUR ADVICE

Studies have shown that water can be effective in helping to reduce pain during labour. It has become a very popular form of pain relief with lots of women also going on to give birth in the water as well as labouring in it.

If you want to try out a birthing pool, as long as you are low risk and do not need continuous monitoring then you should be a suitable candidate. You cannot go in a birthing pool if you have had an epidural, have an IV drip, or are being continuously monitored.

—— WHAT TO EXPECT WITH A WATER BIRTH

When you get in the pool, you will realise quite quickly whether you like it or not. For many women, the feeling of the water is relaxing and calming, some describe it like "a big hug". You will be able to move around and find a position that is comfortable to you, perhaps on your knees leaning against the side of the pool, or sitting down with your back leaning on the side.

The midwife or doctor will monitor your pulse and

temperature and the heartbeat of the baby regularly. This will be approximately every 15 minutes or if your contractions are more regular, then sometimes after each contraction.

Some women enjoy being in the pool as their labour progresses, using the water as a form of pain relief, but may wish to get out to have an epidural, or to deliver the baby on dry land. However, many want to stay in the pool and deliver the baby in the water. As long as all the conditions remain good and stable, it may be possible for you to give birth in the pool if that is what you would like to do.

As your labour progresses the midwife may ask you to step out of the pool so that she can see how dilated you are and confirm when you are ready to start pushing. The midwife may encourage you to get into a position that will allow her to see the baby's head as it is coming out. She may explain that she will not help the baby's head out or even touch the baby until it is completely born. Babies have a dive reflex which will stop them from taking a breath underwater, but they should not be startled or this may interfere with this reflex.

When you have pushed the baby's head out you will have to wait for the next contraction before you can push the rest of the body out. This thought may scare you or your partner as you may worry that the baby will inhale water, but their dive reflex will make sure they keep their airway closed until they reach the surface.

With your final push, the baby will come out, and you or the midwife can guide them to the surface and put them straight on your chest. The cord is normally cut while you are in the pool and then you can stand up and get out in order to deliver the placenta.

Some FAQs about water births

—— WHAT SHOULD I WEAR?

Whatever feels comfortable. You could be naked, or wear a bikini top or vest. You obviously do not need to wear anything on your bottom half!

—— DOES MY PARTNER GET IN THE POOL TOO?

This is something you can check with your hospital, but a lot of pools only have room for one.

—— IS IT TRUE THAT IF I DO A POO, IT'S MY PARTNER'S JOB TO FISH IT OUT?

We think this is a bit of a myth, and we've never actually met a birth partner who has been asked to catch a poo and scoop it out. But there is a first time for everything!

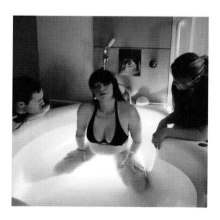

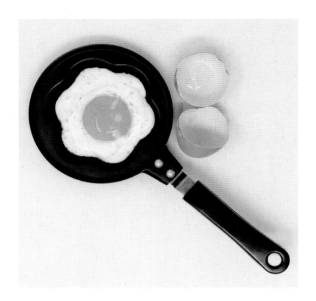

About back-to-back babies

Dr Rebecca Moore @drrebeccamoore
doctorrebeccamoore.com

My second child was born back to back or occipito-posterior (OP).
It hurt in a different way from my first birth. The pressure in my lower
back was huge. It was very strong and intense. I felt like I wanted to
push from very early on in my labour, almost from the very beginning.
I thought "Oh great, I must be fully dilated and ready to push" but
of course I wasn't! I found gas and air and being in water helped
me. I needed to stand and rock, I did not want to be lying flat at all.
The midwife gently pushed against my lower back for a while which
felt good.

 I want mums to know that the pain was different but not awful.

I want mums to know that you can birth vaginally with a back-to-back baby. I didn't tear. I didn't bleed. Lots of women have positive and lovely back-to-back births. One of the midwives with me that day beamed at me afterwards and said, "Wow you had an OP baby, he came sunny side up!" This made me laugh. Then she made me the best cup of tea ever. Bliss. I feel proud to have had a positive OP birth.

—— OUR ADVICE

Around one in ten women have a back-to-back, or occipito-posterior (OP), baby. This means that the baby is positioned on its back inside you, with its head facing skywards, rather than the more favourable position which is where their head is facing down towards your bottom.

A back-to-back baby can be diagnosed by an examination of the tummy or a scan, or by an internal examination if you are in labour. It is often not diagnosed until labour begins. Having a back-to-back baby can sometimes make early (latent) labour longer and more painful. This is because your contractions will need to work harder to soften, thin and then open your cervix. Because the baby's head is not in an ideal position, it is not putting pressure on the cervix to help it with the job of widening. Your contractions will also need to work extra hard to try and get your baby into the right position. This can often be really exhausting and sometimes demoralising if you had not anticipated being in pain before active labour begins.

The position your baby takes in your womb is mostly beyond your control. Some experts believe that there are certain exercises you can do that can encourage your baby to move into a more favourable position, but there is little evidence to show that this works.

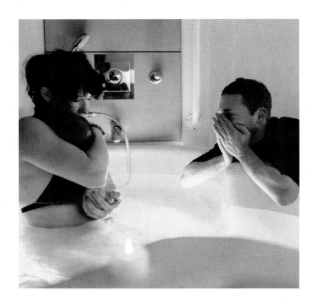

Hypnobirthing can be so powerful

Siobhan Miller @thepositivebirthcompany
thepositivebirthcompany.co.uk

When I gave birth to my first son, I was uninformed; I knew nothing about the physiology of labour and I was frightened. I felt out of control and at the mercy of the medical team. When I was pregnant with my second son, I found hypnobirthing and it changed my life. I went into labour understanding my body and how it worked, and armed with practical tools I could use to help me remain calm and relaxed throughout. Knowledge really is power!

My labour was fast but I focused on my breathing and

visualisations. I got in my little zone and I used positive affirmations to remind myself that I could do this. People tend to talk about how many hours their labour lasted but nobody tells you that surges (contractions) last around 60 seconds – and you can do anything for 60 seconds!

The moment I gave birth to my son I felt euphoric! Never have I been more present in a moment. He was passed between my legs and I brought him up to my chest beaming. I felt invincible.

Every birth is different but hypnobirthing teaches you that it's not the mechanics of how birth happens that matter most, but how the mother feels during the experience, because it's the feelings that last a lifetime.

—— OUR ADVICE

Hypnobirthing encourages you to think and talk about labour and birth in a different way – to help you relax and feel more positive, calm and in control about the whole birth process.

Although it cannot take the pain away, it aims to help you control your emotional reactions to pain. This should keep your stress hormone levels down, which in turn should help increase your endorphin and oxytocin levels which could help you to have a better labour. Endorphins are your happy hormones and oxytocin is the hormone that helps your womb contract and help get the baby out.

You can start practising relaxation techniques at any time in your pregnancy. You can take a physical course which is often done over a few days, or there are courses which you can download and do in the comfort of your own home.

Even if your birth does not go as planned and you end up having an emergency caesarean section, having the ability to stay calm and not panic is a real bonus.

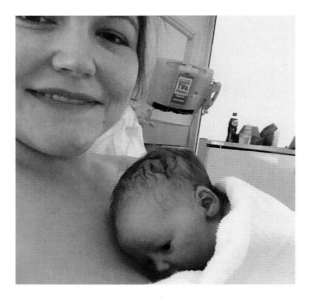

An epidural can be part of a painless and positive birth

Laura Hadrill @laura_hads

17 hours into labour, I finally made it to a delivery room. "You can have an epidural now," someone said. I was terrified of the idea, but I was tired, and the thought of some time to regroup was welcome, so I agreed. In they came, an astonishingly chirpy team, I suppose because everyone is always thrilled to see them. I was contracting so it was hard to stay still, but eventually they managed to site it. I felt a cold trickle spread round my back and then . . . the RELIEF.

I could think, speak, make jokes, laugh, pee (not all at the same time). I slept for the first time in two days.

When I got to 10cm, I stopped hammering on the top-up button quite so aggressively and began to feel an intense pressure in my back and pelvis. I was able to kneel up and use the feeling to push. I was as mobile as I wanted to be. Right at the end, the baby's stats went a bit squiffy so a lovely consultant came in with a ventouse and I finished pushing my son out with some help. I had a 1st-degree tear with a couple of stitches (none of which I felt) and went home the same day. I wouldn't hesitate to have an epidural again.

—— OUR ADVICE

An epidural provides the most effective form of pain relief possible. It works by blocking pain-transmitting nerves that supply the uterus without seriously affecting your motor function (the use of your arms and legs). It is a very safe procedure with less than a one in 10,000 risk of serious problems.

It is normally only given when you are in established labour – which will be confirmed by one or two examinations by a midwife or doctor. Established labour is usually confirmed when your cervix is more than 3cm dilated.

The epidural has to be administered by an obstetric anaesthetist and involves inserting a small plastic tube or catheter into the epidural space in the back, which is outside the spinal cord. A local anaesthetic injection will be given first to numb the area before the epidural tube is inserted. Once inserted, it may take 10–20 minutes to become fully effective and the catheter/tube is left attached so that top-ups can be given regularly as required, by you or by the midwife. It may give complete pain relief and in 90–95% of cases is very effective.

In theory, an epidural can be inserted any time in labour but if labour is going very rapidly and you are almost fully dilated it may be a good idea to consider another form of pain relief or see if you can continue without pain relief, as having an epidural very late in labour can reduce sensation and you may not feel the urge to push, which may slow things down. Having an epidural also increases the chances of needing an assisted delivery, as if you don't feel the urge to push, you may not push as effectively.

You will need a catheter to drain your bladder while the epidural is in place because you will have no awareness of your bladder filling up, which can stretch and damage it. You will also need an intravenous drip to keep you hydrated and to correct your blood pressure if it drops or rises.

Some women can remain mobile during their epidural, but most are more comfortable on a bed as your legs may be weak due to the lack of feeling in the bottom half of your body.

If I ask for an epidural does it mean I failed?

—— DEFINITELY NOT!

There is no shame at all in opting to use pain relief.

If it is managed well, an epidural can be used as part of a very positive and painless delivery. To optimise the chances of a spontaneous delivery (without forceps or ventouse) you need to listen to your midwife or doctor about the timing of your epidural top-ups, especially in the second stage of labour, before pushing. Some women are able to push effectively with a total block but many cannot feel to push and may then need assistance in the form of ventouse or occasionally forceps.

Generally, the more you can feel, the better you can push, and the more epidural you have had, the less likely it is that you will be able to push the baby out. There is a window of opportunity that a good midwife or doctor will be able to try and steer you towards – the idea is to try and let the epidural wear off sufficiently for you to have enough sensation to push, but not so much that you are in uncontrollable pain. The skill of the midwife or doctor and the understanding and agreement of you and your partner are essential for this to work.

A common observation of women, their partners, doctors and midwives is the complete change in atmosphere after an epidural is given. Women report feeling totally normal as soon as the epidural starts working. If before you have been writhing in pain, unable to speak or concentrate on any questions you are being asked, you may well find you can now relax, sleep, watch a film, chat to your partner or midwife and you may feel that you regain control of the situation.

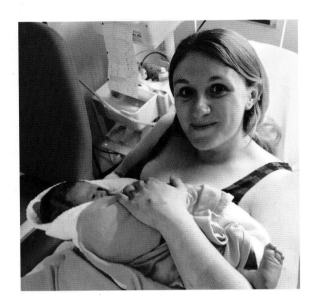

Being induced is not as scary as it sounds

Emily Cocozza @emilycocozza

Nobody tells you that being induced can be a really positive experience. I was induced because my pesky baby didn't want to come out after 13 extra days. I wasn't dilated at all when I was induced, and my cervix was still very much posterior. I had the pessary at midnight and was lucky enough to be able to go home. Contractions started about 2am and I ventured back to the hospital at 11am where I was very much in labour. I had some gas and air and used my TENS machine, stood up and moved loads and gave birth to a 9lb 8oz baby at 9pm with no other interventions.

I was really nervous about induction, but it went so smoothly – just trust your body. If you don't want to be induced, however, you have every right to refuse after being fully informed of the benefits and risks, and just have regular monitoring of you and the baby if you want to. There are always options.

—— OUR ADVICE

About 20% of women may need to be induced. This may be because of concerns about the baby and/or the mother and sometimes a combination of both. The most common reason for induction is to prevent prolonged pregnancy (over 42 weeks).

The word "induction" strikes fear into the hearts of so many women and we think this is unnecessary. An induction does not have to be a horror story. It can often be a really good experience and the more favourable your cervix, the more likely this is. Please have a chat with your midwife or doctor about this if you are worried.

Any decision made about being induced should be made carefully after a suitable consultation with a midwife or obstetrician. This discussion should include a full explanation of benefits to mother and baby and also the risks.

—— HOW DO YOU INDUCE LABOUR?

There are several ways of inducing labour and the method used will depend very much on how favourable your cervix is. This is determined by an internal examination to see if the cervix is soft, stretchy, open and baby's head is down – these are favourable conditions. If it is firm, long and closed and the head is high then induction of labour may be more difficult as conditions are not so favourable.

See overleaf for more detail on the different methods.

How do you induce labour?

—— 01: MEMBRANE SWEEP (SWEEP)

A membrane sweep (often just called "a sweep") is normally considered before any drugs or invasive procedures are undertaken. This involves an internal examination by the doctor or midwife who will attempt to insert a finger through the cervix and try and separate the membranes that surround the baby and stimulate local hormone release. When the cervix is favourable this may work in one in three cases. If the cervix is unfavourable this is unlikely to work. This is normally done between 40 and 41 weeks. It can be an uncomfortable procedure that can produce a small amount of bleeding but it is very safe.

—— 02: PROSTAGLANDIN

The most common way for labour to be induced is using a prostaglandin gel, tablet or pessary, which is inserted into the vagina. Some women will go into labour after the first dose, but it is not unusual to need two or three applications at six-hourly intervals. The gel will usually produce some significant contractions and your baby's heartbeat should be monitored carefully for the first hour or so after the use of the prostaglandin. Some women respond quickly and others may have a delayed reaction and a few (especially where the cervix is unfavourable) may not progress. After the initial monitoring, you will be encouraged to stay mobile but near the hospital.

—— 03: ARTIFICIAL RUPTURE OF MEMBRANES

This is an alternative method of induction but can only be performed once the cervix has started to open. It is also often performed to speed up a labour which is progressing slowly. It is often combined with the use of Syntocinon. Once the cervix is open enough, the membranes can be artificially ruptured by a midwife or obstetrician using an Amnihook. The Amnihook, a long thin stick that resembles a crochet hook, can look pretty scary. The procedure can be a little uncomfortable but it should not hurt. You might like to use the gas and air while this is being done.

——— 04: SYNTOCINON

If the use of prostaglandin is thought to be unsafe or unsuitable, or if the cervix is very favourable but contractions are not very effective, then a combination of membrane rupture and an intravenous drug called Syntocinon may be used. Syntocinon is a synthetic form of the hormone oxytocin. Once this drug is used, it does require continuous fetal heart monitoring using a CTG (cardiotocograph) so you will stay within the hospital and sometimes on a bed. With the use of Syntocinon, labour may be more painful than if it has started naturally, so it can be a good idea to opt for some effective pain relief like an epidural.

——— WILL INDUCTION INCREASE MY CHANCES OF NEEDING A CAESAREAN SECTION?

Contrary to popular belief, it is now well established that induction of labour actually reduces the chance of an emergency C-section and reduces by 50% the chances of unexpected serious problems with the baby (compared with those that are not induced).

——— CAN I ASK TO BE INDUCED?

Induction of labour at the mother's request can be safely done from 39 weeks but only in the right conditions and if there is a careful assessment of the pros and cons. The more favourable the cervix, the more successful the induction is likely to be.

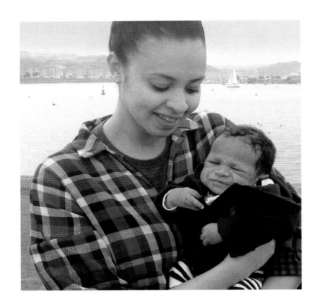

You might tear

Precious Mealia @precious1ne

My surprise pregnancy at 22 was a blur. My local antenatal course was full and so I did my own research on what to expect. I seemed to have skipped over vaginal tears in my research and the advice I received from other mums did not feature this very common side effect of giving birth.

When the time finally arrived, my son was eager to enter the world and after a short active labour he arrived, a tidy 6lb 12 oz. A quick internal examination revealed I had a few tears and the small episiotomy they carried out would need fixing too.

Following an hour and a half of having my legs in stirrups, and some local anaesthetic while eating buttered toast, it was tidied up but caused weeks of pain and a trip to the GP to trim a wayward stitch. Sitting on my breastfeeding pillow was my new favourite place and walking long distances brought on an intense searing pain. The stitches were checked regularly by the midwife at home and although the stitches dissolved, the sensation stayed for around a year.

I have friends who suffered 4th-degree tears requiring surgery months after giving birth, whereas another gave birth to a 10lb baby without tearing. Sometimes there is not much you can do to prevent it, but it's something that mums-to-be should be aware of.

—— OUR ADVICE

Approximately 80% of women who have a vaginal birth will experience some damage to the perineum, and of those 60–70% will need stitches. The good news is that with a quick diagnosis (which can often include a finger stuck up the bottom to feel around!) and some reparative stitches, things should feel better within six weeks. However, if you experience any pain, redness, fever, extra bleeding or it is affecting your sex life or just life in general then please seek help immediately. Treatment is available and no one should suffer in silence.

2nd-degree tears are the most common. 3rd- and 4th-degree tears happen in approximately 5% of vaginal births.

See more about the different kinds of tears overleaf.

The different kinds of tears

——— 1ST-DEGREE TEAR

This is on the inside of the vagina only. It is unlikely to give any problems either at the time of delivery or later. It rarely needs stitching unless there is heavy bleeding. Healing is usually very straightforward.

——— 2ND-DEGREE TEAR

This involves the vagina and the bridge of tissue between the vagina and the anus, called the perineum. This stitching usually requires either local anaesthetic or gas and air, or the topping up of an epidural if one is in place. You will usually have to be in stirrups while this is done and it can take anything from five to 40 minutes. You can normally still hold the baby or hand it to your partner or midwife.

——— 3RD-DEGREE TEAR

This means that the tear has extended into the sphincter of the rectum. This will need to be repaired carefully to prevent any future problems with the back passage, such as incontinence. This repair is normally done under optimum conditions, which are in an obstetric operating theatre. It may seem like a big performance at the time and a complete annoyance after a difficult birth, but it's worth it. You will need careful follow-up appointments with physiotherapists and a postnatal gynaecologist.

——— 4TH-DEGREE TEAR

This is just like the 3rd-degree tear but the tear actually goes into the rectum. Repair is as above but a little more detailed and longer.

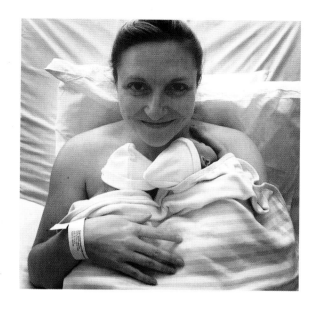

What to expect with a planned caesarean section

Alison Perry @iamalisonperry
notanothermummyblog.com

I was scheduled in for a C-section so that my twins could be delivered safely. I wasn't prepared for how strange it would feel to walk into the operating theatre. There were so many people in there (more than usual, since I was having twins), some of them busy preparing for the procedure and looking very serious, and some of them giving me a reassuring smile and making small talk.

    I've had a few operations, under general anaesthetic, before, but being awake while surgeons cut you open on the other side of a flimsy blue curtain is just surreal. "They've made the first incision," a kind and chatty anaesthetist told me. But it was so hard to believe her. I couldn't feel a thing! People say that it feels a bit like someone's doing the washing-up in your torso, and it's the best way to describe it. You can feel some kind of sensation – a bit of pulling here and a bit of tugging there – but nothing you can really put your finger on.

My whole body shook during the procedure – the kind anaesthetist assured me that it was just my body reacting to the epidural, but I wasn't so sure that it wasn't from fear.

Then I watched as a baby, and then a second baby, was held up in the air (*Lion King* style) at the end of the operating table, for me to see. Just. So. Surreal.

—— OUR ADVICE

Caesarean sections can feel very strange and sometimes scary if you do not know what to expect. However, understanding as much as you can about the procedure can help to allay any worries that you might have.

What can you expect with a planned C-section?

Most elective (planned) caesarean sections are carried out because of increased risks to mother and/or baby. The procedure is nearly always performed under an epidural or spinal anaesthetic so that the mother is awake and can enjoy the experience (as far as is possible). If you are having an elective caesarean you will usually be given a time and date for the operation. This will be as close as possible to 39 weeks.

You will normally meet your surgeon and anaesthetist before you go into the operating theatre. Your partner can accompany you if he or she wishes but will have to wear surgical scrubs, hat and shoe covers. There will be approximately eight to ten people in the room – including an anaesthetist and their assistant, the surgeon, who will be an obstetrician, and their assistant, your midwife, a scrub nurse and their assistant, and in some cases a paediatrician and perhaps a medical student . . . and very shortly, your baby!

The baby's heart will be monitored briefly with a hand-held CTG device, and an intravenous drip will be set up in the back of your hand to keep you hydrated and control your blood pressure. You will have a clip on your finger to measure oxygen saturation in your blood and some sticky pads on your chest to monitor your heart rate. The anaesthetist will insert the epidural or spinal block which will normally start to work within five minutes.

You will usually be tilted to the left with a cushion below your right buttock – this is to take the weight of your womb off the major blood vessels that take blood back to your heart. If this is not done then your blood pressure may drop, which is not good for you or the baby.

It may take up to 30 or 40 minutes for all the conditions to be suitable for surgery. Your pubic hair will be shaved up to a few centimetres above your pubic bone and a catheter inserted to allow you to empty your bladder while you have the epidural in.

A screen will be erected in front of you so you do not have to see the surgery. The surgeon will make an incision about 10cm wide across the stomach about 3cm above the pubic bone. During the procedure you will not feel any pain at all, but perhaps a sensation that has been compared to someone doing the washing-up in your stomach or rummaging in a handbag! Sometimes you will feel some pressure as the obstetrician or assistant helps to deliver the baby's head. If you like, you may request to have the screen dropped so that you can see as the baby's head is delivered.

—— WHAT TO EXPECT AFTERWARDS

From incision to your baby being born is usually very quick, usually about five minutes. After the baby is handed to you, the surgeon will spend 30–40 minutes sewing you up.

After your operation, the first four to six hours of care will be in the high dependency area to look out for complications such as bleeding. You will also have received some intravenous antibiotics to help prevent infection, some blood-thinning injections, and white stockings to reduce the chances of blood clots.

Your catheter and intravenous drip will be removed after 12–24 hours. You may have a drain to remove fluid from the abdomen, which will also be removed after 24 hours.

Stitches will usually be removed after four or five days, or if they are dissolvable then they will not need removing. A feeling of numbness around the scar is normal, and this will usually wear off over the following days or weeks.

You will usually bleed, through your vagina, in the same way as a woman who has had a vaginal birth. You will probably also experience the same after-pains as your uterus contracts after the birth. You may also experience pain from the wound and also from trapped abdominal wind. The hospital will offer you pain relief and you should take this if you are in any discomfort. Our advice is to say "yes" to all the drugs offered for pain relief for the first 24–48 hours, and then take them as required.

The average length of stay in hospital is three days and usually by day 5 you will be feeling better.

Also, see our top caesarean tips on pages 102–3.

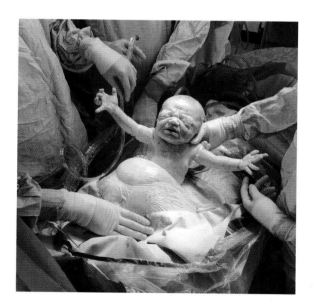

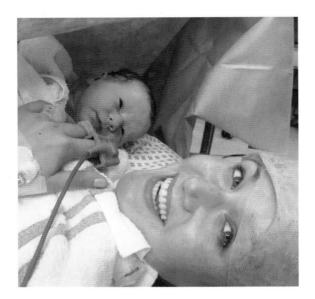

An emergency caesarean section can feel scary

Janey Carey @mummy_buddy
mummybuddy.org.uk

About ten hours into my labour the midwife pressed the "red buzzer". I'd heard about this during my antenatal course (thankfully) and knew that a thousand people were about to come charging into the room. Suddenly my body didn't feel like mine. My limbs were pulled around like a rag doll, the chaos, the prodding and poking with a sense of urgency.

I can still hear it now . . . "Mrs Carey, your baby isn't happy. We are going to get him out immediately." The anaesthetist was incredible. He took my phone to record the birth as he didn't think my husband would make it in time. Those moments after were scary. Helplessly lying there thinking that I was going to lose my baby. Sheer panic. But before I knew it, I was in the operating theatre, the medical team were so reassuring and put me at ease and then my husband stumbled through the door just in time to see our beautiful baby boy arrive!

I can vividly remember the relief from hearing him cry. I remember kissing him. I remember the bright lights. I remember feeling really tired and confused . . . but our baby was healthy, he was fine, he was perfect . . . it was all over.

Has it put me off having another? Oh no way – I'd do it all again in a heartbeat!

—— OUR ADVICE

Around one in three to four women will give birth via caesarean section in the UK so it is important to learn about this and all the different ways of giving birth so there are no nasty surprises in store!

Emergency caesareans are usually carried out because of concerns about the baby or mother's condition.

EMERGENCY CAESAREANS MAY BE DUE TO:
- fetal distress – often diagnosed by changes in the baby's heart rate
- prolonged labour and/or "failure to progress" where you are stuck at, say, 6cm
- bleeding
- going into labour with a breech presentation (where the baby's head is not pointing down)
- problems with the placenta or umbilical cord
- other health concerns about the mother

Most emergency caesareans are performed within one to two hours of the decision, and under certain circumstances some can be done within half an hour or even quicker.

In most cases, though, it is not as dramatic as the "emergency" part of it sounds, as there is usually no immediate risk to the mother or baby.

The procedure will pretty much happen as with an elective or planned caesarean section, which is described on pages 95–9.

TOP CAESAREAN TIPS FOR YOU
AND YOUR PARTNER:
(these may be especially helpful if they are squeamish!)
- if there is a metallic/silver light above the operating table, don't look up at it unless you want to see a reflection of the operation behind the screen
- be prepared for a gurgling noise when the incision is made, and also when the nurse uses the suction pipe to suck up some of the blood and fluid
- the smell of blood can seem strong and can be unpleasant for some people
- amniotic fluid when mixed with blood looks like lots and lots of blood and can seem scary to someone who has not seen it before
- the baby may not cry as soon as it's born, but usually cries within one or two minutes
- you cannot hold the baby until the cord has been cut
- stitching you back up again takes between 30 and 60 minutes and you or your partner can hold the baby while this happens
- drugs will be given to you during and after the operation to prevent infection. Blood-thinning medications will also be administered to prevent clotting, and a variety of other

medications are given to provide good pain relief and keep the uterus well contracted
- sometimes the anaesthetic drugs, the antibiotics, the drama and the surgery itself can make you feel nauseous, frightened and occasionally a little shaky or shivery. This is not unusual and usually disappears after the operation; it is helped by seeing and holding the baby, and some appropriate TLC from your midwife, nurse, anaesthetist and partner.

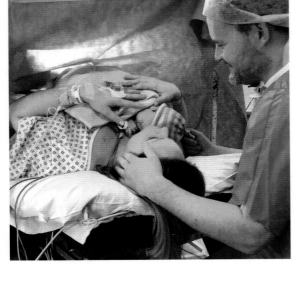

You could request a gentle caesarean section

Lorna Hayward @mrshhayward

After two traumatic emergency caesarean sections, I never believed I would feel so proud of the birth of my third and final baby.

In the lead-up to my third birth I heard people talk about a "gentle section" – a calm, unobtrusive and controlled approach to an abdominal birth. That was what I hoped for and what I worked towards for the rest of my pregnancy. I was able to meet my obstetrician, anaesthetist and midwife before my birth, so at least four out of the ten people who would be in the room were known to me beforehand. I cannot tell you how invaluable that was.

When we arrived in the operating theatre, I felt calm and safe. Everyone in the room introduced themselves. My husband Jamie was with me throughout, holding my hand while the spinal was administered and there was a lovely sense of calm.

And so, at 10.55 on Thursday 8 November the screen was lowered, and we watched as our baby was born. It was utterly mind-blowing. It honestly took my breath away. He was handed from the obstetrician to the midwife, and straight onto my chest. Another wish was that he wasn't "cleaned" and so he was placed on my chest as he should be – vernix 'n' all!

While the screen was raised again and I was sutured, our music was playing, Reggie was on my chest and we were in such a bubble it was unreal. I felt empowered, proud, in love and safe. It was healing, magical and everything I had hoped my birth would be.

—— OUR ADVICE

A "gentle caesarean" can be an amazing experience for the mother, birth partner and the medical team involved. It can be done very safely, with no extra risk to the mother or baby, but needs a little extra thought and preparation from all those involved.

If you know you will be having a C-section and you feel you would like to have a "gentle" caesarean then this is something you need to bring up with your consultant. Ideally you would have a few sessions with your surgeon, anaesthetist and midwife to explain how the whole event will unfold, to make you familiar with the environment.

It all depends on there being no complications with the mother or baby's condition. At no stage will "best practice" be sacrificed. With a little extra planning, teamwork and attention to detail, a routine operative delivery can be transformed into a wonderful and unforgettable experience.

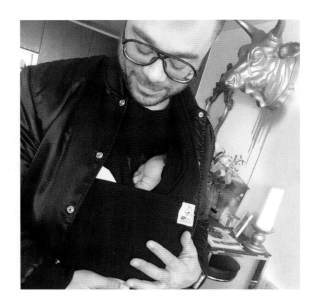

Your birth partner is so important

Rachel Simms @raysimms5mua

I've never loved this man more. Thank you for staying by my side during the labour and breathing me through every single surge, even if you did make me want to giggle when you missed a few numbers!

Him just being there and being 100% present throughout the whole experience was amazing. He left my side twice – once to go to the toilet and once to re-wet my flannel! He made me feel safe, secure, calm and like I could do anything. He kept me focused on meeting our baby boy rather than actually giving birth, if that makes sense? A lot of people asked me if I was sure I didn't want a friend or my mum or sister – a female who had experienced birth – to be there with me, but I'm glad that I had Shane by my side as my cheerleader and coach. I honestly couldn't have asked for anything more from him!

Thank you. I couldn't have done it without you and I appreciate you and all that you do for us.

—— OUR ADVICE

Your partner might just be indispensable during your labour. Lots of people imagine their partners to be useless, as they are so often portrayed in Hollywood movies. Like a spare part, hanging around being annoying and not knowing what to do. Looking at the wrong bits for too long, coming over all queasy, fainting or saying the wrong thing at the wrong time.

Maybe that is why male partners often haven't been invited into the delivery room in the past and instead directed to the pub until it's all over? Well it's not fair, because actually they can be totally amazing and complete naturals. If your partner understands the birth process and your wishes, and wants to be there and to play a part, there is no reason why they can't be the most incredible birth partner you could imagine!

CONTENTS

Postnatal:
the early days

The first few days and weeks can sometimes pass
in a blur of cuddles, nappies, bodily fluids and streams
of visitors. Taking it easy is paramount and lining up
some support is vital. Don't race to be up and at it
too quickly. Take it slowly while you adjust to the huge
changes that have occurred for you, inside and out.

This chapter explains what those early days may
feel like and reveals so many useful things that
Nobody Tells You . . .

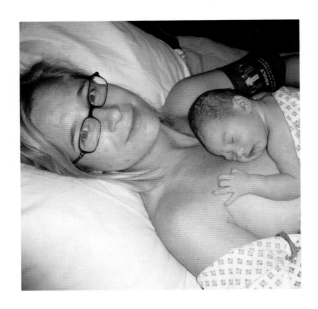

It's not always love at first sight

Deenie Lewis @deenie19

I do find it weird when women describe having their babies as "the best moment of their life" – seriously?! With all the pushing and screaming and pooing and swearing at the father? And then the moment you meet your baby and there is supposed to be an overwhelming surge of love for them and angels sing and you cry happy tears.

Am I the only person who found labour a bit of a drag? And the emergency C-section 36 hours later not that enjoyable? So when the nurse asked if I wanted to hold my new baby I was

exhausted and grumpy and found myself responding, "Not really."
When my baby was born she had that weird cone-head thing so
they had put a little woolly hat on her and my thoughts on first
seeing my baby were "Eurgh, I really don't like her hat." So within
seconds of being a mother I had rejected my baby and mentally
slagged off her outfit. I felt massive disappointment about the
whole encounter but, actually, this is only one day, one moment,
and I have felt the overwhelming surge of love for my child ever
since. So bollocks to the Instagram birth, it's what happens every
day after that is truly motherhood.

—— OUR ADVICE

Please don't worry if you don't feel that rush of love you were
expecting. Birth is exhausting and often painful and sometimes
traumatic, and it's not surprising that we don't all feel that
enamoured with our babies as soon as we see their little faces.
If you are feeling completely worn out, perhaps shaky, or even
nauseous, you may not feel you have the energy or ability to hold
your newborn. And that's ok! Your partner or midwife can hold
your baby while you catch your breath and take in the enormity
of the situation. Your bond with your baby will not be affected
by taking this brief pause so don't worry that not immediately
adoring your baby makes you a bad parent.

We should also add that some babies are very funny-looking
when they have just been born! They may be a bit more wrinkled/
blotchy/unattractive than you had imagined but regardless, you
will still feel the love.

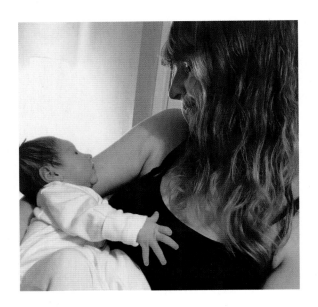

You might feel like you have run a marathon

Rinn Purvis @mama.tinny
mamatinny.simplesite.com

After over 96 hours in labour . . . I thought that giving birth would signal an end to all the aches and pains. I was wrong.

Stitches, after-pains, the pure aching of your muscles. Muscles I didn't even know I had! In this picture (one of the rare candid pictures taken by my fiancé) I'm gazing lovingly at my tiny five-day-old baby . . . what you don't see is how I'd spent all day crying about how exhausted and sore I was and the fact I was pretty much bed/sofa bound.

The thing is, giving birth is JUST like running a marathon. It's long, and tiring, but the end result is amazing and so worth it, but if you are in pain then you need to treat yourself like you've run a marathon. You need to sleep, rest, fuel your body with food and concentrate on getting to know your newborn better! Don't worry if others are out and about in ASDA six hours after giving birth. That's great they feel so good after! However if you don't feel ready then that's fine too.

—— OUR ADVICE

Everyone needs some time to recover from childbirth. Whether your baby is born via caesarean section or a speedy textbook vaginal birth, it is hard work on the body and the mind and you will definitely feel the effects. Some women get a surge of adrenaline and find the whole experience so exhilarating that they are unable to sleep and just want to be awake and taking it all in and racing off to the supermarket! Others are exhausted and are able to switch off and take time to rest.

It is sometimes hard to try and guess how you will react, but take the cues from your body and your mind. If you are feeling exhausted and weepy then please try and get some sleep. If you are feeling good then of course feel free to get up and about, but do also remember not to push yourself. The postnatal period is a long-distance event rather than a sprint. Try to make sure there are no undue extra pressures on you during this time, let the usual chores slip a bit and understand that it is ok to let the laundry pile up and to eat ready meals for a while and accept help from family and friends.

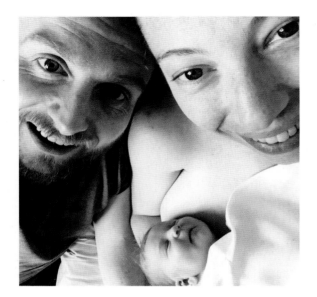

About the postnatal ward

Amelia Evans @hellobabyantenatal
hellobabyantenatal.com

I am a midwife, so I'm well aware of what postnatal wards can be like. They are very busy places, with a high turnover of patients, the constant soundtrack of crying newborns and buzzers going off, and excited visitors flocking in and out.

   The staff are under a lot of pressure. If you work on a postnatal ward your bum hardly touches a seat all day and you're lucky to get a lunch break, yet you can still feel you've not provided great care. This is sad – as this is often a time when mums are at their most vulnerable and hormonal, and need lots of emotional and physical support, as well as practical guidance on how to care for their new baby.

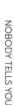

What can you do to make that hospital stay more manageable? While it's not always possible to get a private room, I'd always encourage people to go to a hospital where partners are allowed to stay. Bring something comfy for partners to sleep on and in (otherwise they might just be upright in a hard chair all night). Make sure to send them out for decent food for the both of you. Remember to utilise all the on-tap advice and pain relief, and try to enjoy the lack of cooking/cleaning/washing-up and the restricted visiting times!

—— OUR ADVICE

We think it is important that there are no nasty surprises in the postnatal period so it is a good idea to be prepared for your time on the postnatal ward. We do not want to frighten anyone or put them off staying overnight on the postnatal ward because if you need support for yourself or your baby, then this is probably the best place to be. BUT sadly a lot of women are not very complimentary about the time they spend on these wards.

Common complaints about postnatal wards are that they are understaffed, noisy – with babies crying, loud conversations and other people's visitors – and they are very warm. It's horrible to hear, but the shared loos are often not as clean as they might be, so we advise taking some anti-bacterial wipes with you.

They are usually extremely busy and lots of women say that they are pleased to get out as soon as possible. They are, however, a secure environment where mothers and babies can get the support they need, sleep, rest and concentrate on recovering from childbirth.

Be prepared. Don't expect a 5-star hotel! It's warm, it's loud and it's likely that you will be woken during the night and early in the morning by babies crying, women talking (sometimes on their mobile phones in the night!) and breakfast being served. Remember this is a temporary stay, you're not moving in.

The midwives will likely be stretched and you may need to be pushy to be heard. If your baby is not latching on, you can ask that they are checked for tongue tie. If you are struggling with breastfeeding or want to be shown how to hand express then ask, ask and ask again.

And if you are feeling unwell, experiencing what appears to be an abnormal amount of bleeding or have any other cause for concern do speak up – loudly if you have to! Your and your baby's health are paramount.

Please don't discharge yourself early even if you are having an awful time. The doctors and midwives do know what they are doing and it is important that you and your baby receive all of the necessary checks and care before going home.

You might feel lonely and scared – perhaps it's your first baby, perhaps your partner or family cannot be with you or you experienced a difficult labour. Try reaching out to the other mums on your ward. Just talking can really help and you won't feel so alone. They are in exactly the same boat as you.

Essentials for the postnatal ward include:

Toiletries as if you were going on a minibreak!

Earplugs – don't worry, you will still hear your baby if they cry

2–3 nighties with straps or buttons down the front for breastfeeding (if you are planning to breastfeed)

The Mother of All Pants (postnatal pants) (available from amotherplace.com)

Maternity sanitary towels

Flip-flops or slippers for trips to the loo – the floors can be a little skanky at times!

Anti-bacterial wipes in case the toilets are not as clean as you would hope

Cash for food and drinks

Phone/tablet and charger

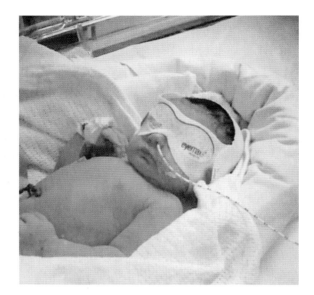

You might not go home the next day

Hollie Storr @honestlyhollie

My waters had ruptured four days before my labour began and I not
only had an infection that had passed to my baby but I was
developing sepsis. My baby was whisked away by the paediatric team
from SCBU (Special Care Baby Unit) for a cannula and IV antibiotics. I
was also started on antibiotics and told I had at least a week's stay in
hospital. I was so confused and scared. None of the books prepared
me for this, and I had read many! All of my friends were home the
same day with their bundles. Why was this happening to us? I felt
helpless and just sobbed at not being able to even hold my baby.

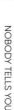

God bless the NHS. The SCBU nurses, doctors, midwives – they were amazing! They worked so hard to help my baby and thankfully three days later she was showing signs of improvement. Three days later we went home. It wasn't the birth and postnatal experience I had imagined. It affected me for a long time afterwards and I felt quite cheated out of the "normal" experience. It's made me very nervous of having another baby as I'm scared it could happen again, even though the chances I know are slim. I guess you cannot prepare for every eventuality but I would advise any woman to approach her birth and the postnatal period with an open mind.

—— OUR ADVICE

It can be a shock to find out that your baby is unwell and then to realise you will not be taking your baby home as quickly as you thought you would.

How long you spend in hospital after giving birth will depend on individual circumstances, the mode of delivery and the condition of you and your baby. Even if you had a very straightforward birth and are ready to go home in six hours, you may find that your baby needs some extra medical attention.

It may not feel ideal and it may be very nerve-wracking, but rest assured, the hospital is the best place to be if either of you is unwell.

If you have an uncomplicated vaginal birth and you and your baby are well then you can usually go home the next day or even, sometimes, after six hours, if you really want. If you have a caesarean section then the stay is usually around three days, although some hospitals are offering some women a fast-track discharge, so if you are feeling well and healing nicely and are confident you have proper support, you may be able to go home after 24 hours if you want.

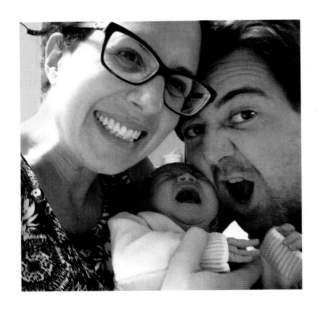

You might be home
before breakfast!

Charlotte Inston @dickieinston

My firstborn arrived at 00:47 and after a few stitches we were told we could go home, just a couple of hours after our son arrived and straight from the delivery room.

It seemed other-worldly; just a few hours before, we had left the house as two and were returning as three, having been shown the very basics of nappy changing and breastfeeding. There was a wonderful calmness to being back in our own space, having a quiet cup of tea and a shower in my own bathroom. Then we began to call our nearest and dearest to tell them the wonderful news. While some expressed pure joy at our news, I was not prepared for the extent of the negative remarks surrounding our very brief hospital stay, suggesting a mandatory 24 hours minimum were required in order to be decent parents. Comments ranged from the extreme "your baby could have died", suggesting only hospital air keeps them alive, to despair at the state of the NHS kicking a new mother out so soon, refusing to accept this may have been a personal choice.

Would I have such a hasty retreat again? Well, I did with son number 2 who arrived at 03:57 and we were home a couple of hours later to find our eldest still in his PJs having just got up. And that first cup of tea at home was wonderful!

—— OUR ADVICE
You just don't know how your birth will go, how you will be feeling, how your baby will be doing or how busy the postnatal ward will be. But if you had a complication-free birth, you're feeling well and confident, your baby has fed and there are enough available staff to deal with your discharge, you could be home as soon as six hours after giving birth. For some women and their partners that may sound like too much too soon, in which case, don't worry, you will not be sent home against your wishes! For others, it's what they had been hoping for and they are delighted to be home in familiar surroundings as soon as possible.

If you are very keen to get home, yet the conditions are not in your favour, please do not be disappointed or get frustrated. Enjoy the support offered at the hospital and relax, you will be home soon.

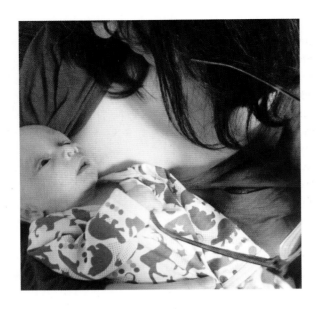

About premature babies and special care

Natasha Morabito @natasha_morabito

Nobody tells you what it's like to have a baby in special care. When you're feeling scared and all the other mothers on the postnatal ward have their babies with them and you are only allowed to go in every three hours for a cuddle and an attempt to feed a very very sleepy premmie, it's strange. It's disconnecting. You aren't sure the baby is really yours. You miss out on bonding, but when you're there with them it's so precious.

Nobody told me how crushing it is to be asked which formula you want your baby to be fed with (through a nasogastric tube) when you'd planned to breastfeed from birth. Nobody told me how weird and tricky it was to collect colostrum by hand-expressing and catching every drop with a 10ml syringe. How awful it felt if you missed. But also how it takes your mind off other things.

Nobody told me how quiet it is in the special care baby ward. They don't really cry because they don't have the energy. They're all tiny, but not as tiny as the ones in NICU. You're lucky you made it to 35 weeks. A lot luckier than some.

The delight you feel when your baby opens his eyes. He doesn't do it much, so it's like a gift. The moment when you realise the "eff eff eff" noise he's making is his attempt at crying. The wrinkly tortoise neck where there's no fat, just skin and bone. But in your eyes he's the most beautiful and perfect baby.

Nobody tells you about the benefits either – two weeks in special care means a nurse on hand to help you learn to breastfeed when you don't know what you're doing. Not just five minutes with a harassed midwife with a knitted boob. I got to sleep and I had time to heal from my caesarean. Nobody told me how terrifying it would be to finally be left in charge and take him home.

—— OUR ADVICE

It can be a real shock to find that your baby needs to spend some time in special care. However, it's not that uncommon because around one in ten babies may need some special care. If they are having trouble breathing, feeding, keeping warm or are unwell then this is the best place for them to be. You will be given lots of emotional and physical support by midwives and nurses and most people look back on this time as being nerve-wracking but also very special.

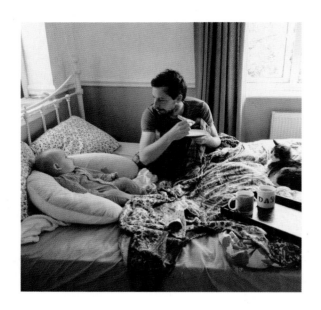

Coming home with your baby is surreal

Emilie Sandy @a_mothers_gaze
emiliesandy.com

When you get your baby back from the hospital for the first time, your cat can appear to have doubled in size. And you suddenly understand what responsibility really means!

No longer was "responsibility" merely a case of just putting down a bowl of biscuits, or clearing up the odd fur ball: no, the game had changed. We realised that straight away when we greeted our (now) giant cat with our tiny baby boy in hand.

You won't remember all the useful things you have been told.

My midwife had told me to try feeding my baby lying down in the night because it is less disruptive. Did I remember this amazing advice? Nope. Instead, I insisted that my husband bring our small sofa into our bedroom for me so I could sit up straight to feed our baby, along with a feeding pillow that had to be "perfectly" placed for the optimum position. What a load of faff, right?

We forgot about the outside world. It was snowing and cold outside at the time and we became hermits and literally lived in our bedroom, eating three meals a day in the same room – because it felt safe and warm. My husband became my butler, chef and nanny while I fed our baby (he still is my butler, chef and nanny six years on . . . but, shush).

—— OUR ADVICE

It can feel very strange to return home for the first time with an extra person – and a brand new person too! Sometimes just hours old. You might not know quite what to do with yourself, and with them. Don't worry though, you'll work it out. As long as you remember to feed them and feed yourself, change their nappies, change yours (!) and make sure you both get a bit of sleep, you will be fine.

New babies need feeding, changing and keeping warm and you need time to rest and recover, and those are the most important things. If holing up and forgetting the outside world for a while feels good, then go for it! You will work out your own way of parenting in no time.

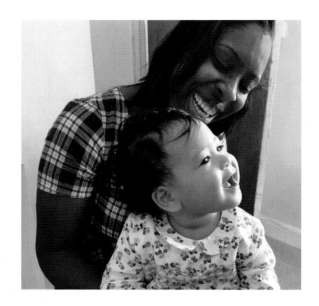

About your first poo

Olivia Manley @mrslivmanley

We were having one of those lovely moments cooing over our new baby when I felt an urge. I told my husband it was time for "The Poo". I waddled to the bathroom and attempted to lower myself to the toilet. I had read all the horror stories and was shitting it!!

I'd had a ventouse delivery, which meant that she had been dragged out by a sweaty but kind obstetrician with a large and brightly coloured plunger, so I was feeling particularly battered. I sat on the seat and quickly decided that I would have to do this standing up. I leant against the cold wall tiles, said a short prayer and relaxed. Apparently certain parts of me weren't quite working so I strained a little and ripping pain shot right through me and I shouted my husband's name. He ran in holding the baby. He was very kind and said lots of lovely encouraging words. Holding the baby, he took my hand, I held on to the wall and, encouraged by my audience, I very, very slowly took my first poo as a new mum. It was painful, it was messy but it was done.

—— OUR ADVICE

Every woman is nervous about her first poo after giving birth. But it doesn't have to be that bad! To put it very simply, the softer the stool (poo), the easier it will be to get out and the less strain it will put on your abdominal muscles and perineum (the area between vagina and anus). To keep your poo soft you must try and stay hydrated, which is easier said than done in those first few days.

Giving birth is dehydrating, the postnatal ward is hot and sweaty, breastfeeding is dehydrating and certain medications you may be given can also make you a bit constipated. So try and drink lots of water and eat fresh fruit. Kiwi fruit are a natural and mild laxative and eating a couple after you have given birth can be a great idea to get things going!

Don't worry if you don't need a poo for a while. You may have emptied your bowels before or during your birth, and you probably won't have eaten much during your labour, so your first poo may not be due for a day or two.

If you suffer from constipation then a product like Fybogel which contains ispaghula husk should help. You can get this over the counter or on prescription. Please talk to your midwife or doctor.

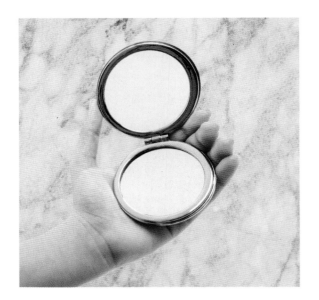

How your fanny might look and feel

Annie Ridout @annieridout
annieridout.com

After giving birth to my daughter (forceps, tearing, episiotomy), I remember hobbling to the toilet on the postnatal ward to do a wee. As I wiped, I wondered what on earth had been attached to my vagina. It was as if there was a bulbous pad attached to it. It hurt, and was unrecognisable to touch.

I got home and decided to have a look at it in a hand mirror. It was a bit of a mess, to be honest. Later that day, I thought I had an infection so I went to the hospital. As I walked in, three-day-old babe in my arms, I burst into tears. I told the nurse I thought I had an infection in my stitches and that I had no idea what had happened to my vagina. She inspected me, slowly and gently, and then got a pen and paper. She drew a vagina and marked where I'd torn and where they'd done the episiotomy. There was no infection, she said. Once I understood what had happened down below, I felt less scared. I cried again, because she'd been so kind.

The next day, the swelling had massively reduced. A week later, it looked just as it had pre-birth. I thought I'd end up with a bucket fanny. I didn't. It shrank back to its normal size so quickly.

—— OUR ADVICE

We think you should avoid looking at your fanny in the mirror for a while. There is not a lot to be gained from having a look immediately after giving birth. Whether or not you had stitches, it's not likely to be a pretty sight in the first few days or weeks and indeed it may never look exactly the same again, but it WILL get better. We suggest having a feel when you're in the bath and you will probably be able to notice any changes – it may feel quite alarming at first and this may or may not encourage you to have a look.

We suggest that you wait until you have healed before getting the mirror out for an inspection! And when/if you do, please don't freak out if you don't like what you see; it takes time for everything to go back to normal.

The vulva and vagina usually heal very quickly and usually within six weeks they will be back to their new normal. If you experience any increase in pain, redness, extra bleeding, fever or things seem to be getting worse rather than better, please speak to your midwife or GP immediately.

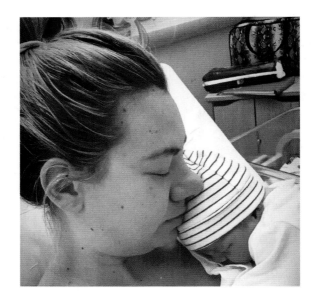

You can say "NO" to visitors

Megan Shaw @tobyoliverandme
tobyoliverandme.com

With my first baby the first few weeks of his life are a complete blur with visitors traipsing in and out fondling this new little human. I would sit watching, smiling and nodding along to conversations, just wishing they would all go away.

Second time around I'm very aware of how important my mental and physical health is. I'm doing what's right for me and my family, and I want to enjoy every second, I need to take things really slow. I want to study every little inch of him and really get to know each other. I really want to enjoy it this time. I want to give our family time to adjust; this is my second baby and I'm so aware of how much of a massive change this is going to be for our family.

Napping in the afternoons, staying in bed all day, not rushing around worrying about if there are any clean mugs for visitors to have a brew, if the house is a mess or if I've washed my hair. None of it matters in the grand scheme. Those tiny baby days pass by in the blink of an eye, I fear with Toby that I missed them, and I'm not going to allow that to happen this time. I deserve this time, I deserve a happy and positive experience.

There's plenty of time in the weeks that follow for visitors and they will be welcomed with open arms once Dan is back at work and Toby is back at school and I'm all alone with a new baby, I'm sure of it! But those first few weeks – they are ours.

—— OUR ADVICE

You must not feel bad about controlling the number of visitors you receive. It is such an exhausting time and although it's lovely to be able to show off your new baby, it is so important to rest and take it all in yourself. Visitors can often be demanding with their time and aren't often appreciative of how tired you may be. Many outstay their welcome, eat all the snacks and don't even make their own cup of tea.

If you want some time to yourself with your new family then please be honest and explain this and tell people that you are really excited about their visit, but ask if they could come in two weeks when your partner is back at work and you will really appreciate the company and support. If you feel too bad to do this then get your partner to break the news. Real friends will not mind.

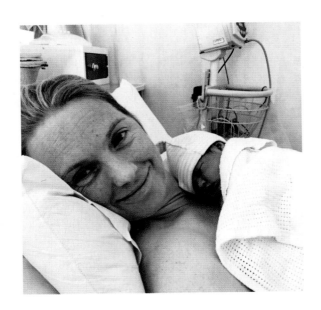

Night sweats feel disgusting!

Camilla Richardson @pinkstormsocial

I had no idea that for three weeks after having a baby I would have to sleep on a towel because I was drenching my bed sheets every night! Nobody told me the windows would need to be wide open, that it would be freezing in my bedroom when I went to bed but still I would wake up drenched in sweat with the sheets stuck to me and my hair dripping like I had just got out of the shower!

Nobody told me that my night sweats, combined with overflowing breast pads and sanitary towels and a little one waking every two hours would send my husband next door into the spare room and culminate in such long, lonely and unsettled night-time hours.

Uuughhhh!! One of the most unpleasant and unsexy parts of the postnatal period! As if you aren't already excreting enough bodily fluid, your sweat glands want to join in and douse you in buckets of perspiration. RANK! It's really bloody horrible when you wake up soaked in the middle of the night and you are flailing around in the dark trying to work out if you're covered in milk, blood or what?!

—— OUR ADVICE

Night sweats can feel really horrible and can disrupt your sleep, but rest assured they are perfectly normal. They are a result of a combination of changes in your hormones and your body ridding itself of excess fluid it has taken on during pregnancy. We suggest sleeping on a towel with a sheet between you and your duvet, and with a spare towel and sheet by your bed. If you wake up wet then simply remove the towel and sheet and replace (it may happen more than once in a night).

Some women like to sleep with ice packs and another idea is to have two separate duvets so that you and your partner can control your own temperatures. If your night sweats are accompanied by fever, swollen breasts or flu-like symptoms then visit your GP straight away to check for mastitis or any other sign of infection. If they continue beyond six weeks it is worth mentioning this to your doctor too.

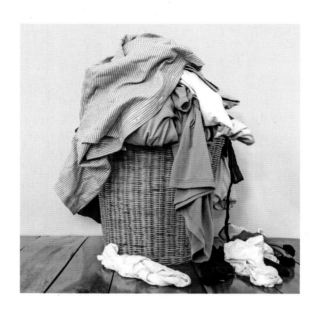

About piles

Anon

I was ready for the piles of laundry . . . but it was the ones hanging out of my bottom that really took me by surprise!

Nobody told me that piles are a common side effect of pregnancy and childbirth. Apparently all the extra blood flowing round places where the skin is quite thin makes them common. And nobody, absolutely nobody, told me that breastfeeding can make you constipated which makes your piles even worse as you strain to do a poo. So bad it hurts to sit down. Which is kind of what you need to do while you're feeding.

So having just got over childbirth and the total lack of dignity entailed with that, you're then straight back to the doctors, showing your arsehole to some poor unsuspecting GP. But as ever with the NHS, she was great. Totally matter of fact and totally understanding. And with some super-powerful cream and a quarter of a watermelon a day, it all improved quickly. And just to clarify, you eat the watermelon to keep you regular and get your fluid intake up. Don't try sticking it anywhere else or you'll really be in trouble.

——— OUR ADVICE

The medical name for piles is haemorrhoids – these are swollen veins around your bottom (anus) and feel like lumps which can be sore, itchy and cause bleeding when you go to the loo. You can get them when you are pregnant, giving birth or breastfeeding or you may even have had them before. When you are pregnant you may get a bit constipated, and when you are straining to do a poo, the added pressure of your uterus and the baby can force some of the blood vessels in your anal canal to pop out.

You may also develop piles as a result of pushing out a baby. During the pushing stage it is possible to push some blood vessels out of your bottom.

Some women can even get piles for the first time in the postnatal period, often while breastfeeding. Breastfeeding can make you a bit dehydrated and this can cause you to become constipated which can make you strain on the loo and push them out. Or you can just get piles because your forebears had them and you are genetically predisposed to developing them!

See overleaf for our top tips for managing piles.

Piles: what can I do?

It sounds disgusting, but when you're having a shower or bath or when you're cleaning your bottom, have a feel – if you can feel anything poking out, then gently use a finger to push it back in. Make sure you have cut your nails!

There are lots of over-the-counter creams and ointments you can get in the chemist – happily they are on the shelves so you don't have to ask the pharmacist for them if you are feeling embarrassed.

If things feel painful then suppositories and cream together are a good idea.

Using moist toilet tissues after going to the loo can help.

Warm baths and cold compresses are a real relief if you are feeling sore or itchy, especially after giving birth.

And if things are really really painful and sitting down becomes an issue, you may need a small, inflatable donut-shaped cushion or rubber ring for a week or so.

If your piles do not get better after the birth of your baby and continue to be a nuisance, then it is best to see your doctor who might suggest treating them with an injection to shrink them, or perhaps even removing them in a quick and easy operation.

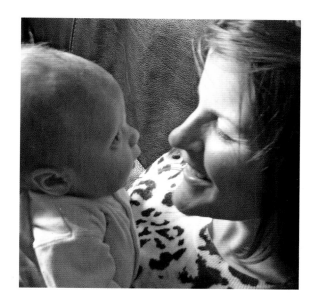

The fourth trimester is just as important

Amy Ransom @amyransomwrites
notebooksformums.co.uk

I wish I had discovered the glorious fourth trimester before my third baby. It's a crucial period for you both – the first 12 weeks of your baby's life and your new life as a mum where you mimic your baby's environment inside the womb, outside – and allow yourself to make the transition into motherhood, gently, slowly and lovingly. Where you cut yourself some serious slack (and some cake). And focus on the most important thing of all: replenishing yourself after nine months of pregnancy and labour. And getting to know your baby.

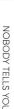

Because, while it might seem obvious that this is what you should do, the reality is that lack of sleep, a comment from another mum whose baby is sleeping through, or a book you read, might make you feel you should be doing better.

Lower your expectations. Accept that you will feel up and down. Allow yourself to feel however you feel in any given moment.

In the first three months, at least, anything goes. There is no right or wrong so don't tap into any worries or let them spiral into catastrophic thoughts.

Keep reminding yourself, "I've just had a baby."

You are doing amazingly.

—— OUR ADVICE

We seldom educate ourselves about and make plans for the postnatal period. Often called the fourth trimester, it's just as important as the other three trimesters and we need to prepare ourselves for it as well as we do for those. So many of us have all the gear and no idea! The nursery looks Instagram-ready, the drawers are filled with the cutest babygros, the bags are all packed, the books have been read and the hypnobirthing done, yet we haven't made any plans for what is actually ahead.

We need to be honest with each other about what it is like and accept that it may not be all cuddles and beautifully photographed moments. We need to find a way to be realistic without scaremongering. You need the emotional and physical support for what is often the hardest part of the whole journey – settling in and finding a new normal.

There is no right or wrong way to behave in those first few weeks, but there is no doubt that taking it easy and accepting help are good things to do.

How to prepare for the fourth trimester

Think about your support network. Who can you count on for emotional and physical support? Who will come and push the buggy around the block while you have a nap? Who can you call when you are having a bad day?

Do you have a "policy" in place for visitors? Will it be a free-for-all or no visitors for the first two weeks?

What will you be eating? Ready meals? Takeaway? Does your partner cook? Can you fill your freezer in advance? Have you mastered online grocery shopping?

Try not to commit to anything too stressful too early on. Friends will understand if you can't make their events.

Where will you get support with breastfeeding if you need it?

What groups and centres do you have near you that run mother and baby activities?

If you spend a little time thinking about some of these things before you give birth then you will be in good stead for the weeks and months ahead. This is not an exhaustive list, but it's a good place to start.

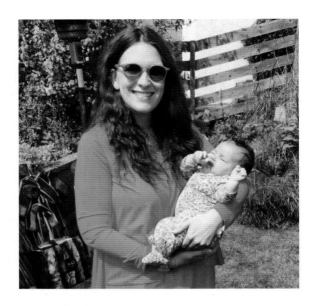

Your 6-week check might be underwhelming

Jennifer Jones @jczreid

As with pretty much every part of having a baby, I was obsessed with asking everyone what to expect at my 6-week check: should I take the baby? Do I need that funny-sized red book? Should I shave my legs?! I ended up imagining a sort of competency-based job interview, and went armed with prepared answers like the doctor had the power to let me be a mum or not.

It turned out to be a huge anticlimax; my doctor asked me about three things: my mental health (fine), my physical health (fine) and my sex life (non-existent!). There was no examination or blood test or multiple-choice questionnaire as I had been led to expect. It took about five minutes and I left feeling a bit "Is that it?".

And yes, I did shave my legs just in case.

—— OUR ADVICE

Traditionally, the 6-week check used to be a bit of a milestone and something that new mums looked forward to. It was a chance to chat to your GP about your birth, how you were coping and to get some advice on contraception, pelvic floor and perhaps weight loss. Today, GPs are so overstretched this often does not take place. In some parts of the country you will only get a 6-week check if you ask for one. In some places you may be invited for a 6-week check and find you are in and out within five minutes. This may not be a big deal if you had a textbook birth and both you and the baby are doing well.

However, if you had a complicated birth, your baby is not feeding well, you are not feeling great and perhaps need some physio, then you will need more time and a more thorough consultation, and not all women seem to be getting this. If you are not invited for a 6-week check and would like to talk to someone about your birth and yourself and your baby then we would suggest that you call your GP. You may want to book yourself a double appointment if you feel that you have more than one issue to discuss, as it can be frustrating to be cut short and sent home because the GP does not have time.

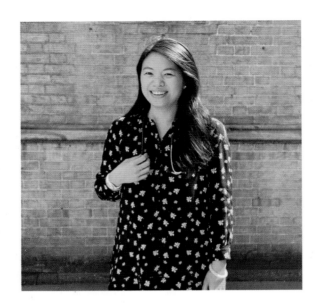

Being a doctor doesn't make you a better mum

Dr Stephanie Ooi @the_gp_mum

I've had so many people say that I must know what I'm doing because I'm a doctor but, to be honest, it couldn't be further from the truth. Parenthood has been a whirlwind so far, an exciting and exhausting journey. There was nothing that could have prepared me for it. There are so many aspects that I had no clue about at the beginning and am still learning about. Medical school didn't cover how to leave the house on time with a baby (answer: never!), how to deal with "poonamis" or what to do if your toddler has a tantrum in the supermarket. The only thing that might have been slightly helpful was doing night shifts. #sleepdeprivation

However, I definitely think being a mum has made me a better GP. At least, I hope so. There's a new appreciation and understanding when a parent brings in their child and they have had a rough sleepless night. In addition, occasionally I can share some tips that I've tried and vice versa. It's solidarity at its best.

So the answer is no, I'm certainly not a better parent than anyone else because I'm a doctor. I am learning as I go along and doing what feels right, just like everyone else.

—— OUR ADVICE

It just goes to show that you can read all the books, take the courses, even qualify as a doctor and there is STILL so much that will take you by surprise on this journey. It is comforting to hear that even doctors, midwives, nurses and nannies – people who spend their professional life working with pregnant women, babies and caring for others – still don't necessarily have it nailed when they come to start their own family. Like many things in life, the theory is often quite different from the reality.

Get ready for parenthood to teach you a whole new skill set: multi-tasking (doing a poo with a baby on your lap while doing an online food order), prioritising (sleep or Netflix?), humility (no one escapes being hit by a liquid yellow poo), patience (leaving the house on time will be a distant memory), realistic expectations (sleeping for three hours straight feels like a week at a spa). If and when you head back to work after having a baby, you may well find these new skills give you a headstart in the workplace.

CONTENTS

Postnatal: your mind

The postnatal period is often the bit that comes as a shock. We've been busy concentrating on the birth and the cute babygros for our new arrival and suddenly . . . BOOM . . . our world changes overnight! For the better of course, but there may be some bumps along the way.

For many mums, the newborn phase is dreamy. But for some, it can be more difficult than they anticipated. Your birth experience, hormones, lack of sleep and changes to your dynamics at home can sometimes affect your psyche, so it is good to know what to do if things don't feel quite right.

This chapter focuses on the emotional side of the postnatal period. The stories all offer hope and positivity to those who need it and we make sure there is nothing that Nobody Tells You . . .

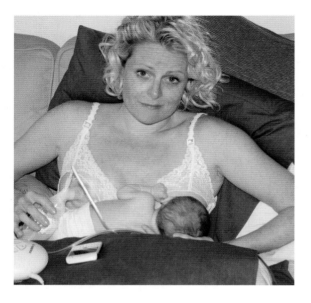

We all get the baby blues

Becca Maberly @amotherplace
amotherplace.com

On days 1, 2 and 3 I thought I could conquer the world! I was euphoric, excited and so happy. But on day 4 I crashed.

I was up all night feeding, I couldn't work out why my son was crying. My husband was chipping in with unhelpful things like "Have you fed him?", my boobs felt like they were going to explode at the seams, I had soaked through my favourite PJs with blood. I had a feel of my bits in the bath and nearly passed out in fright at what I felt. The doorbell had gone again and woken my son and now I had a hallway of visitors! The house was a tip and we didn't have any biscuits to offer them and then I remembered my husband was going out that night to "wet the baby's head" for the second time that week.

And so on day 4, I cried. Everything was too much.

My husband ushered the visitors out. He pushed the baby around the block and I ate, had a shower and a nap. And when I woke up I felt so much better!

───── OUR ADVICE

We all get the third- or fourth-day blues. You're probably going to have a cry and it's ok! It's normal. In fact, if you don't cry then that's a bit strange. We can guarantee that every glamorous celebrity mum you can think of would have had a cry around day 4. Even with all the money in the world, all the support you could ask for, and a hair and make-up team on call, you can't escape the hormone changes and huge emotional wave that hits you.

The baby blues occur after a sudden drop in your oestrogen levels just after you give birth. Your oestrogen levels, which have been super high during your pregnancy, drop more than 100 fold in the first three or four days after your baby is born, and this can make you feel teary.

SO WHAT CAN YOU DO?
- let it all out – just cry as long as you need to
- have something to eat
- get someone to take the baby out for a walk in the buggy or in another room
- sleep
- when you wake up, you will feel like a new person!

The baby blues usually last a day or two. If you feel that your symptoms are not easing and you suspect that your mood is a more serious issue, then please speak to your midwife, health visitor or GP.

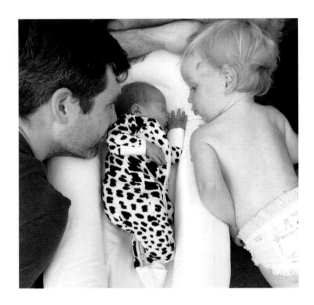

You will worry about your baby

Olivia Dudleston @olivia.dudleston

I've always been a pretty relaxed parent, however I found that the responsibility of parenthood hit me when I least expected it . . . in the middle of the night! During the relentless night feeds, where I couldn't be sure if I was asleep or awake, I had a constant fear that I was going to fall asleep and suffocate my baby. I would wake up in the night frantically patting down my husband thinking our baby was in the bed and we'd squashed him.

The first time it happened I managed to also send my husband into a panic and he duly started helping me flap the duvet around, but with subsequent episodes he quickly learned that I was just half asleep and having a nightmare. With my first baby I would wake up most nights for over a year with the same fear and neurotic behaviour. It hasn't been quite as bad second time around, but I do still occasionally panic that the little cushion I like to cuddle in bed is in fact my baby, and also still dream that my toddler has gotten out of his cot and is asleep somewhere in our room where he isn't safe. I guess the message about SIDS subconsciously had a real impact on me!

—— OUR ADVICE

It is so normal to worry. We all worry about our unborn baby when we are pregnant, and then the real worrying begins when we first bring our babies home. Your worries will become less intense over time as your baby gets bigger and you become more confident. But the worry never really stops completely. You stop worrying about one thing and move on to another! Is that a rash? Is it a heat rash or meningitis? Is that cough just an ordinary cough or is it pneumonia? Is that cry for attention or is he in pain? And then as they grow older – will he be ok at nursery? Was it mean for me to make him eat his broccoli even though he insisted he hated it? Should I have read him an extra bedtime story when he asked? Am I an awful mother? Am I doing enough?

You know what? If your parents are still alive, no matter how old you are, they probably still worry about you! It's just a natural part of parenthood.

If you or your partner are concerned that you might be worrying excessively then please do speak to your GP or midwife.

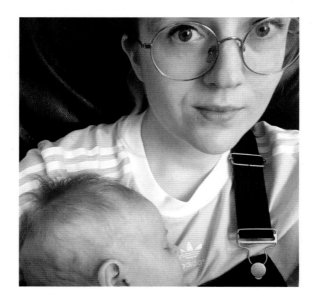

Bonding with your baby isn't always immediate

Danii Kedik @daniikedik_design

My son was born by emergency C-section and had difficulties when he was born. He was rushed to SCBU (Special Care Baby Unit), so I didn't get to meet him until he was 12 hours old. We never got the beginning I envisioned and was told was so important.

I immediately knew a love I had never felt before, and would do literally anything for him. But he was like a puzzle I couldn't solve. I was frightened to hold him – what if I disconnected a wire? Or didn't support his head? What if he hurt my wound as he was so damn heavy?

I tried to breastfeed him but he was not getting enough milk and cried constantly. I cried with him.

I couldn't understand this baby. Why couldn't he do it properly? The sound of him crying made me resentful. He was stealing my body and my sleep. Then followed crushing guilt for feeling that way about my beautiful baby boy.

I gave up breastfeeding and worked through some serious mum guilt. Within a few weeks, without realising, the unbreakable bond I imagined had been formed.

I had been putting myself under too much pressure. I forgot to be present in the moment and let the bond grow. Like any relationship, it needed a little time, patience and work.

—— OUR ADVICE

You don't always feel that rush of love that you hear about. Sometimes you look at them and think "Wow, you're amazing and you seem very nice" but you don't always feel that strong pull on your heart that you might have been expecting.

If you have had a difficult pregnancy or birth, or a tough postnatal period then this can help explain why bonding is not always immediate. But for some women, there is no real reason behind this initial inability to bond. You mustn't feel guilty about not feeling this intensity of love for your baby; it is more common than you think, but people are a bit embarrassed to talk about it as they worry it makes them look like a bad mother. There is usually no cause for concern and the maternal love that you have been looking for will usually creep up on you and you will suddenly realise how in love you are with your new baby.

If, however, this feeling continues for more than a few weeks and you are worried that you may be suffering from postnatal depression or perhaps suffering from the emotional after-effects of a traumatic birth, then please speak to your health visitor or GP.

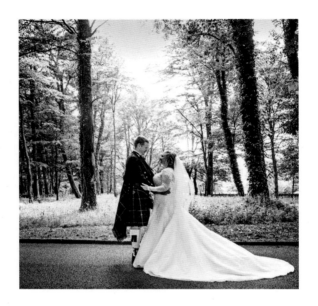

Your relationship with your partner will change

Emma Phin @emma_phin

I remember when I was pregnant the first time, a friend casually mentioning something about "You'll find your own routine and then your husband will come along and mess it up". I remember thinking that wouldn't happen to us.

Well once the sleep deprivation really kicked in after I'd had the baby, my once lovely, thoughtful husband couldn't get anything right. I felt like I was the only one who could and the responsibility was overwhelming. My husband desperately wanted to help but I felt that I was the expert. We were arguing about daft things like bins not being emptied or him putting the baby down five minutes late for her nap. I remember thinking how are we going to make it through this? All I could see was pictures of other happy families on social media. I felt like we were failing but I now know others were going through the same things.

For us, communication was key, and understanding it's ok to be on two different pages for a while. Second time round we knew what to expect. We were happy to accept that our relationship might need to sit on the shelf for a bit, but it wouldn't be forever and we've worked a bit harder to appreciate each other this time round.

—— OUR ADVICE

Your relationship will change and there is no doubt about it. We are not saying it will change for the worse, hopefully it will be for the better, but either way there may be a period of adjustment.

A brand new, noisy, demanding little human has arrived to live with you forever and it takes time to find a new rhythm and way of doing things. For heterosexual couples, no matter how much we wish that we could have complete sexual equality, this is one time where the woman usually bears a lot of the emotional and physical load. For women, things change dramatically overnight. It is the woman who has given birth and if you want the baby to be breastfed, it is the woman who will be feeding the baby.

Some partners adapt quickly to the change in home life, others ignore the change, and their social life and professional life continue unaffected. And many are somewhere in between. Either way, for some women, it can be difficult to see your partner head off to work or the pub while you are confined to the sofa with the task of keeping your offspring alive! We are generalising of course, but the change is massive and you should be aware that it may take some time to work things out together.

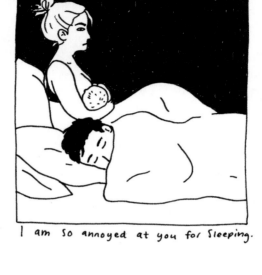

I am so annoyed at you for sleeping.

You might resent your partner

Emma Ahlqvist @fromthepine
emmaahlqvist.com

I often feel annoyed when I see my partner sound asleep next to me, when I am awake at 3am, feeding our child. I know it makes sense for him to sleep so that he will have the energy to tidy up the house and cook me dinner tomorrow, but still I am angry that he is sleeping. I want him to not sleep for the same amount of time so that he knows exactly how tired I am. I want to wake him up because being awake for hours in the middle of the night, feeding a newborn, can be so lonely. I know that he would wake up if I asked him to, but when the morning comes I am happy that he has had more sleep than me because he brings me coffee in bed and cooks me food.

—— OUR ADVICE

This can be so tough and there is no simple solution to offer because everyone's situations are different.

It's hard not to feel resentful that your partner is getting more sleep than you. Many partners are able to snore their way through every night feed which can be so frustrating if you are up for the zillionth time that night. Sometimes you wish they would wake up to provide you with some company, as the night feeds can feel so long and lonely. Sometimes you just want them to wake up and appreciate how heroic and selfless you are (and bring you a drink and a snack). And other times you want them to wake up so they know how absolutely exhausted you are – to share your pain! It's very normal to feel all these things.

If you have a partner with a job that demands that they get eight hours' sleep (brain surgeon/pilot/tightrope walker) then perhaps it is best that they sleep in a different room. If their job is a little more flexible or they can still function well at work with less sleep, then perhaps you can talk about them doing a feed in the night? But if you are exclusively breastfeeding then that won't work.

Some of us are early birds, some of us are late owls, but we all need a certain amount of sleep to function well and stay healthy. There are many things that your partner can do to support you practically and emotionally, early morning or late at night, so we would encourage you to have a think, discuss this and make a plan that works for you.

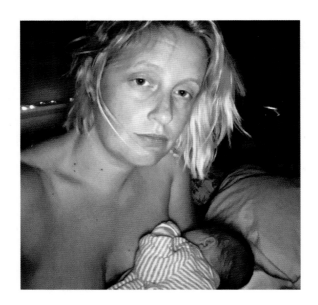

You need to manage your expectations

Cat Sims @notsosmugnow
notsosmugnow.com

Motherhood is wonderful and it's the best thing you'll ever do. It's really bloody hard and it'll test your patience and your strength to the very limits. Every day, you'll be blindsided by these tiny humans that you made and you'll wonder at the crazy magic of it all . . . even if, at that particular moment, you want to put them out by the bins.

Try and manage your expectations. During your first pregnancy, all you'll hear about is what a special time it is and they're not wrong. What they don't tell you is that those first few weeks and months are hard. Really hard.

Here's the thing . . . Aunty Barbara won't tell you about the stitches she had that hurt so bad she had to sit on a rubber donut for six weeks. Your neighbour won't mention the cracked nipples, the blisters, the mastitis. Your mum won't talk about how she spent those early days unable to shower because you wouldn't let her put you down. Your mate won't tell you about the loneliness she felt when everyone went back to work and your work colleague will forget to tell you how her marriage was pushed to the edge with the pressure and the sleepless nights and the total lack of time to commit any energy to the couple they once were.

Those first few weeks are a huge adjustment and you need to give yourself and your family space to do that as quietly and as slowly as you need. So lower your expectations of yourself and then, lower them some more. You've got a whole lifetime to be the best mum you can be . . . right now though, at the beginning, you've just got to figure out what being a mum actually is.

—— OUR ADVICE

Too often we put all the emphasis on the wrong things and too much pressure on ourselves. The Pinterest-inspired nursery becomes more important than organising some postnatal support. The antenatal classes become all about making new friends and less about choosing a good class that will give you honest and realistic advice. The late-night googling and lurking in forums becomes more important than sitting with a trusted friend.

The newborn days are tough, but they do pass quickly, so do what you need to do to make life easier for yourself and your family. No one is expecting anything from you at this time – after all, you have just performed one of life's greatest miracles and deserve a break from performing any others.

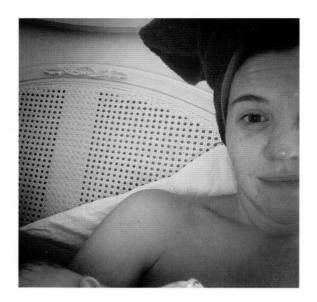

Motherhood is hard

Steph Douglas @steph_dontbuyherflowers
dontbuyherflowers.com

I struggled after my first babies and nine days in it's too soon to
know how this one is going to go, but I have learned that:

- We are our harshest critics and no one is judging us more than
  ourselves.
- This is a phase and it will pass – whether that's the lack of sleep,
  difficult behaviour, the rage at your partner.
- Do everything you can to be kind to yourself because no one
  can look after you better than you. If that's leaning on others for
  practical help, sharing how you feel, going to the doctor, sacking
  off all cooking and cleaning while you rest and nap, or writing a

ten-point email to your partner (when calm) on ways they can help you.
- Surround yourselves with the good ones – the women that get it and get you and will nod along, share their own cock-ups and hold you when you need a cry.

I don't believe anyone doesn't find motherhood hard. In this picture I've just given birth and am feeling elated it's over and he's here safely! Since then I've felt weepy, ragey, giddy, ecstatic, engorged, content and everything in between. It's a rollercoaster, made slightly less terrifying for having done it twice before and knowing this is just how it is.

——— OUR ADVICE

We are trying to raise our babies in a very different world to generations before us. We are more isolated, living in two-bed flats on streets full of people we don't speak to, in different cities from our potential support networks of grandparents and aunts and uncles.

We are the generation of women who were sold the idea that we could DO IT ALL! But it's not true. You can't be a successful businesswoman, supportive and loving partner, domestic goddess, chef, cleaner, organiser, great friend, fitness fanatic, healthy-eater AND a good mother. It just isn't possible! We all need support and whether that is from family or friends or paid help, it doesn't matter, but just acknowledging that you can't do everything and learning to ask for and to accept help is very important.

Try not to be so hard on yourself – let some less important things slide and see how it feels. Don't stress about letting older kids use the iPad so you can have a shower and get dressed, and grab some ready meals so you're not stuck in the kitchen when you could be sitting down and recharging. Leave the laundry and go meet a friend for cake! Your children are loved, fed and warm – you're doing great.

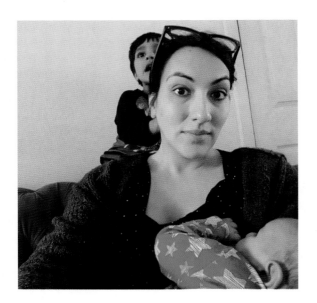

It takes a village

Saima Mir @saimamir (Twitter) @ben_raf_remy (Instagram)
saimamir.com
The Khan published by Point Blank (March 2021)

Motherhood has taught me the benefits of community and the Pakistani culture in which I was raised. The shared burden of raising a child; the postnatal confinement period of 40 days, when women are taken care of, helped to heal and supported with breast-feeding; the eagerly waiting grandparents, ready to deliver hugs and cups of tea... I missed out on all of this. I envy the ease with which couples who have help navigate parenthood.

I'd heard the phrase "it takes a village", countless times throughout my life, but I never really understood what it meant until I had my first child. My childhood was filled with countless cousins, aunts, uncles, alongside my five siblings. So when I made the decision to move to London to be with my husband and start a family, I had no idea how hard it would be.

I had babies that refused to nap, zero help, and no one else to turn to or ask to take the children long enough for my husband and I to have a chat or a cup of tea. My inability to complete a task thanks to all these things took its toll on my mental wellbeing. I could feel myself slipping away. And as the clutter and chaos increased, I began to feel as if I was losing myself, my mind. I definitely did not feel like a good mother.

Seven years on and my sister had moved to London. We'd just returned from a week away, emptied the car, unpacked suitcases, put dirty laundry in the washing machine, and put three grumpy little boys to bed. My stomach growled. I resigned myself to a round of toast. Then, there was a knock at the door. I opened it to find my sister, holding out a large box of homemade chicken curry, and a loaf of banana bread – it was still warm. I wept. My village had returned.

—— OUR ADVICE

Raising a baby is hard; raising a baby without help is even harder. Lots of us no longer live in large, extended family units and many of us do not even live in the same city as our parents. Flats on streets where we do not know our neighbours' names are the norm for many of us, and as a result we often feel isolated and lonely.

If you don't have a family or network of friends to call on for advice and help then the tough times may often feel tougher. So maybe we need to try and create our own villages. Try saying "hi" to your neighbour! Be brave and ask another mum or dad for coffee (yes, it's cringe, it's just like dating). Strike up a conversation in the nappy aisle in the supermarket. Smile at the mum at the swings in the park. Your village is out there waiting for you!

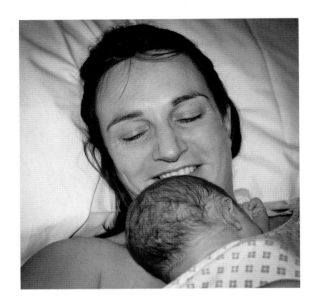

You will find your new normal

Anya Hayes @mothers.wellness.toolkit

I once went to see a friend with her newborn, she was about six weeks in, wide-eyed with sleep deprivation. She said to me, "When does it get back to NORMAL? I want it to feel normal again" . . . and I, chasing my eight-month-old who was about to capsize one of her houseplants in her still pristinely non-baby-proof house, said "Erm . . . soon . . . or . . . never . . .?"

"Normal" is an elusive benchmark for new parents. Is this poo normal? Is it normal that my baby is part koala and will only settle on my body? Is it normal that I miss my baby when I'm not holding them? Is it normal that my baby only sleeps for 20 minutes when the book says they should be sleeping 7pm–7am by now?

Then there's the wishing for "normal life" – humans are routine animals. We like familiarity. We're soothed by patterns. Babies and children bring mayhem. One phase more chaotic, less sleep, the next, peace for a microsecond . . . followed by another disruption. We're constantly reacting, predicting, recalibrating to each new normal.

The very idea of normal has to be fluid once you're a mum. I wish I'd known that initially and just softened into it rather than bracing and waiting for it to be . . . normal.

Early parenthood is a bit like being on a rollercoaster in the dark . . . no idea what's around the next bend. Cling on for dear life, laughing hysterically/screaming . . . and when it gets to the end, AGAIN!! AGAIN!!

—— OUR ADVICE

Things do change, irrevocably, once you become a mum. Your priorities shift overnight. Suddenly this new person is all you can think about, your life revolves around them and just finding the time to brush your teeth and get dressed before midday is an accomplishment! Your body feels and looks different; relationships with partners, parents and friends take on a new meaning; and mixed emotions of anxiety, doubt, joy and extreme happiness will affect your state of mind. It can be a struggle to come to terms with these changes both physically and mentally, to find what we like to call your "new normal".

But it is helpful to try and accept and even embrace these feelings rather than always waiting and wishing for things to return to how they once were. Your new normal is something to celebrate as it marks a new stage in your life where the old you and the new you come together to make a great parent.

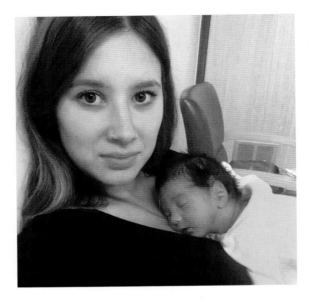

You may feel traumatised by your birth

Annabelle Gray Silks @alovingdoula

My waters broke at 31 weeks and my baby was born at 33 weeks and 5 days, with epidural, forceps and an episiotomy after an agonising 30 hours of contractions. My baby's heartbeat suddenly dropped dramatically, alarm buttons were pressed and people rushed into the room where my boyfriend and I had just been relaxing moments before. I had been on gas and air and the epidural had kicked in nicely.

Suddenly the bed was taken apart and my legs were suspended in the air. I remember looking at my boyfriend and shaking my head as he held my hand. I was told "You are going to have your baby now, Annabelle, push like you are doing a big poo." I did not feel ready.

My baby was literally plopped onto me and I could hardly bear to touch him. He was rushed upstairs to SCBU (Special Care Baby Unit) while I was stitched up for what felt like an eternity. I tried to get some sleep but couldn't stop thinking about what my body had just been through.

I was discharged after two nights in the hospital. I was heartbroken to come home empty-handed. I cried as my lovely boyfriend washed me and got me into bed. The nightmares are getting less vivid and I'm talking about things with midwives, friends and family. We are hoping our son will be home with us in the next week and we couldn't be happier.

—— OUR ADVICE

Whether you have had a traumatic birth, or perhaps just a birth that did not go quite as you had planned and you would like to talk to a professional about your options for your next pregnancy, then you may need some form of debriefing.

A DEBRIEFING SESSION CAN BE VERY USEFUL
IF YOU HAVE EXPERIENCED:
• a long and painful labour
• an emergency C-section
• an assisted delivery (forceps/ventouse)
• a severe tear or cut
• a traumatic experience of any kind during the birth
• your baby had trouble breathing when he/she was born
• you or your baby had a prolonged stay in hospital

165

You may not understand why certain things happened as they did during the birth and you might feel very disappointed when you think about the birth. Talking to a professional about the sequence of events and why things happened can help you to understand your trauma a little better. You may be able to identify triggers and then in turn learn how to cope when you encounter them.

HOW DO YOU GET SOME DEBRIEFING OR EXTRA HELP?

If you are not offered this opportunity by the NHS after your birth then you can request this via your GP and you should be referred. Failing this, you can look for someone to help you as a private patient. If you take this route, it would be advisable to get a proper referral from your GP, preferably with a photocopy of your hospital notes. The photocopy can be obtained, for a small charge, from your maternity unit.

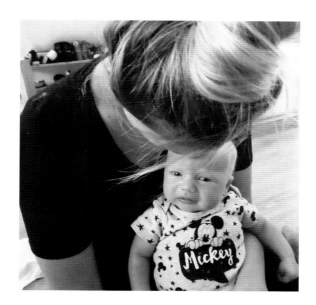

About postnatal depression

Hollie Parsons @whatholliedid
whatholliedid.home.blog

Nobody tells you, you'll be the one to have postnatal depression. I knew the stats but you never expect it to be you.

I went to the classes, read lots of books, had all the apps showing me what size fruit my little bump was each week. The thing I didn't think about was me.

I definitely wasn't prepared for the impact having a baby would have on my mental health. I knew I didn't feel like myself. I cried a lot, resented others and struggled to find joy in any day.

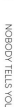

My moment of realisation was when I went for lunch with friends, friends who didn't have babies. My boy had a monumental meltdown and I couldn't settle him. I felt like a complete failure. I ran out of the cafe, into the rain, tears streaming down my face. All very dramatic. At that point I knew I definitely wasn't ok.

If I could give pregnant Hollie some advice, it would be this. Live in the moment, manage your expectations, ask for help and accept it when offered. Most of all, be kind to yourself.

—— OUR ADVICE

Postnatal depression (PND) seems to be more common than doctors have traditionally thought. Recent studies have shown that more than one in ten women suffer from PND, but the exact figure is not known as often women do not report the illness to their doctors and suffer in silence.

THE SYMPTOMS OF PND ARE:

- low mood
- constant exhaustion
- inability to cope
- feelings of guilt regarding your inability to cope or not loving the baby enough
- overwhelming anxiety
- difficulty sleeping
- lack of appetite
- difficulties bonding with the baby
- relationship difficulties with your partner
- low energy
- low sex drive
- social withdrawal (from family and friends)
- crying for no reason

Those who experience three symptoms are considered to have mild PND, five to six symptoms to have moderate PND, and those experiencing more than six to have severe PND.

It is thought to be more common after a bad birth experience or when couples, and women particularly, have unrealistic expectations about becoming a mother or parent for the first time. Sometimes there is an element of lack of support from the partner, friends or family. Women with a previous history of psychological problems appear to be at higher risk. However, not all cases of PND can be predicted, sometimes it just strikes, and with no obvious cause.

If you are suffering from any of the symptoms we have mentioned and are worried that you may be suffering from PND you should talk to your midwife, health visitor or GP as soon as you can and he or she will arrange treatment for you.

If you feel worried that you will harm your baby, then please also speak to your midwife or GP about this urgently. You should not be afraid of telling someone about these thoughts; they will not try to take your baby from you, they will help you to get better.

Treatment is usually very effective and the condition is self-limiting. Behavioural therapy, general support from friends and family, psychological counselling and occasionally medication, all have a role to play. Subsequent pregnancies may also be affected but with good psychological and social support during and after pregnancy, often serious problems can be prevented.

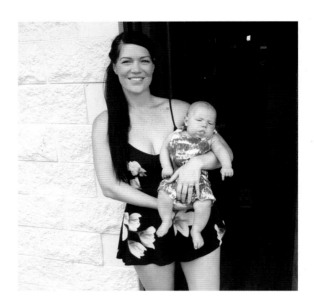

Postnatal anxiety is real

Bianca Markham @bian_ca_nina

This is what a mum with postnatal anxiety looks like. Totally normal, seemingly confident, and going about her everyday business. Except that on the inside, I feel a huge crushing weight on my body, my hands shake, my stomach is in knots and my mind is constantly racing. My baby started sleeping longer and yet I developed insomnia. I felt lethargic, physically and mentally weak, crying all the time as I just couldn't escape myself.

I had to reach out and get help. No one will come knocking on your door and tell you that you need to be looked after. When I was at my lowest point, I went to hospital and was turned away as I just needed to "deal with it". The next day we went to a different hospital, where they took my condition seriously and gave me the help I needed. Michael, my husband, slept in our son Jackson's room so I could sleep for three nights. My mother-in-law has been coming a few days a week to help. Some beautiful friends and family have made meals and given me tonnes of support and between it all, I'm finally feeling like myself again.

I never thought this would happen to me – I'm a strong, confident and intelligent person. Postnatal anxiety/depression is real and it does not discriminate. It's important that mothers talk about this more! Therapy and medication were literally life-savers for me, and hopefully sharing my story can save others.

—— OUR ADVICE

It is very normal to experience some anxiety as a new parent. Anxiety is a normal part of life and it is in fact an important human response designed to keep us and our families safe in dangerous situations. However, if anxiety starts to affect the quality of your life then you may need to get some help.

If you think you are suffering from anxiety then please speak to your midwife or GP and they will be able to help you. Treatment can be in the form of talking therapy, medication or self-help practices like mindfulness and breathing exercises.

Postnatal anxiety is nothing to be ashamed or embarrassed about. It does not mean that you are not a good mother. Luckily, it is spoken about much more now than five years ago and it's important to know that you are not alone.

Common signs and symptoms of postnatal anxiety:

⚡

Feeling anxious, nervous or worried

Feeling that something bad will happen

Feeling tense, stressed or "on edge"

Feeling unsettled

Feeling unreal, woozy or detached

Starting jobs and not finishing them

Unable to sit still and relax

Always on the go

Speaking too quickly

Snappy, irritable behaviour

Drinking or smoking more

Changes in eating habits

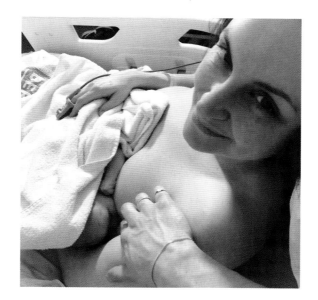

Postpartum psychosis is rare but you should know the signs

Laura Dockrill @lauraleedockrill
lauradockrill.co.uk

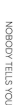

We are all warned about the pain of labour. Of the poo, the blood, the tears and tearing. We've witnessed it on TV. But nobody tells you about what childbirth does to your head. That it could be possible to push YOU out with your baby.

I was a total passenger in my labour. It was frightening, full of panic and featured a whole host of nasty surprises. I was sleep deprived and totally out of my depth. And as I waved goodbye to myself on an operating table, a starving, livid, demanding newborn was thrust onto my chest screaming HELLO.

It was NOT how I imagined it.

At home, I was highly anxious, and couldn't sleep or relax; I was on high alert and scared of something, of everything. I was shrouded with shame and doom. I was feeding my baby but not able to eat myself. I couldn't laugh, I couldn't concentrate. I isolated myself from my friends and family and lost all sense of self. I couldn't sleep even when my baby was sleeping and my symptoms escalated rapidly to delusions, paranoia, mania, dark thoughts and severe low mood. I have never experienced mental health issues before so this was all out of the blue and completely terrifying.

Before I knew it I was hospitalised with postpartum psychosis – a rare and debilitating illness, which is considered a medical emergency. And overnight, my partner became a single dad caring for a newborn.

There has to be more awareness and support in postnatal mental health – I mean, give us a pamphlet at least! My story of recovery is a positive one but it isn't the case for everybody. Many of these cases end in tragedy and it doesn't have to be like this – it is completely treatable.

—— OUR ADVICE

Puerperal or postnatal psychosis is a rare condition affecting around one in 1,000 women. Some women can become seriously psychologically disturbed a few days or weeks after delivery.

If you are experiencing the symptoms (opposite), then you can be a serious risk to yourself, your baby and others around you.

Once suspected, immediate and expert psychological care is needed. With the cooperation of the family, you will usually be admitted to hospital in a secure mother and baby unit for treatment until the condition is improved. Therapy may take weeks or months, depending on the drugs, some of which may affect breastfeeding. Although postpartum psychosis is a serious condition, the vast majority of women make a full recovery.

Some of these psychological episodes can be predicted and prevented, especially in women who have had previous serious psychological problems. If these issues have been highlighted during the pregnancy they can often be prevented by early intervention with drugs and therapy in the antenatal and postnatal period.

There are many support groups all designed to help women and their partners who are suffering from mental illness during or after pregnancy, and these are listed at the end of this book.

Postpartum psychosis is a serious mental illness and should be treated as a medical emergency. Please make it a priority to speak to your GP. If you think you or someone you know is suffering from postpartum psychosis and is in danger of imminent harm, please call 999.

SYMPTOMS OF POSTPARTUM PSYCHOSIS CAN INCLUDE:
- hallucinations
- delusions
- hearing voices
- paranoia
- inappropriate behaviour
- inability to sleep
- you may become out of touch with reality and have no insight into your condition.

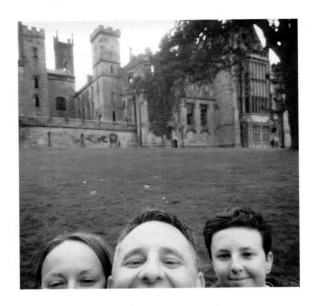

We have to ask dads
if they are ok too

Mark Williams @markwilliamsFMH (Twitter)
#HowAreYouDad

Witnessing my wife giving birth triggered my first and only ever serious panic attack as I honestly thought my wife and baby were going to die. Nothing prepared me for feeling out of control and unable to help the people I love so much.

After the birth I started to feel anxious and worried so much about Michelle even though she was safe. I started to have nightmares thinking both of them had died and even today if I speak about it I can feel the anxiety creeping in.

It put me off sex as I was scared Michelle would get pregnant again as I did not want to risk having any more children. I could never go into a labour ward again.

My personality changed during the first 12 months of my son's life. I suffered in silence for years. Eventually I had a breakdown. Luckily I had some great family support at my crisis point.

I wish I had known that the quicker you get help the quicker you can recover. We must support both mothers and fathers in the postnatal period. The biggest killer of men under the age of 50 is suicide. We have to ask dads if they are ok too.

—— OUR ADVICE

Next to many a mum stands a great partner. They often went through labour too. Sure they didn't give birth, but perhaps they weren't prepared for what they experienced, and this can have a lasting impact.

In many heterosexual, traditional family units, the "modern man" is doing more than ever. He is expected to pull his weight at home. He is taking on more chores and baby-feeding and changing responsibilities than his predecessors, while often continuing to go to work. This can be exhausting and added to a change in dynamics in the home, it can be very disconcerting for many dads.

Our partners can feel the psychological impact of parenthood and can also suffer from postnatal depression. Their relationship has been altered. The mother's focus has perhaps shifted to the baby. They may feel that they have not bonded with the baby as well as the mother, or as well as they expected. This can feel very upsetting and isolating and to compound things, all the attention is on the baby and the mother, and people often don't think to ask the other parents how they're doing. If you are worried that your partner is struggling then please try and reach out and check that they are ok. If they aren't then please encourage them to speak to their GP.

CONTENTS

Postnatal: your body

Our bodies all react differently to carrying a baby and giving birth. A quick look at your own mother might tell you if you're going to be susceptible to stretch marks, but what about all your other bits?

This chapter is full of honest and positive stories from those who have been through it all. There is nothing too embarrassing to share and we know you'll be pleased to hear about all the stuff that Nobody Tells You . . .

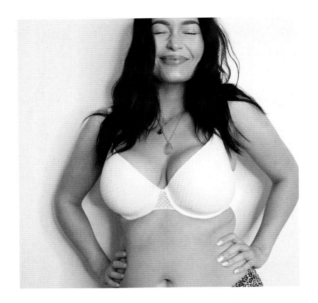

Your postnatal body is amazing

Megan Rose Lane @megan_rose_lane

I'm bigger, softer and squishier than ever before. I'm the furthest I've ever felt from society's idea of perfection. I've cried while trying to squeeze myself into my old clothes, I've contemplated restricting my food and punishing myself in the gym in a desperate attempt to "get my body back".

And then I remember that I'm a miraculous, life-giving human who deserves every single ounce of her own love. I remember that the body I'm so quick to judge and bully just created and delivered my tiny little soulmate, and continues to provide the food for her to grow stronger every day. Without my body I wouldn't be here, and neither would she.

It's a paradox, respecting and loving your body so much for being the vehicle which carries you through life and allows you to enjoy every gift this world has to offer, and then feeling so sad, ashamed and disappointed that it doesn't look the way it's "supposed" to.

Life is so short. You deserve to live fully, to be healthy and happy and joyful and free. Please put self-love at the top of your priority list. Work on it every day, commit to making it the most important goal of all. The more you practise, the easier it gets. And then every time that little voice pops up and tells you that you're not good enough, you can turn around and tell it to go fuck itself. Because you're amazing. No matter what.

—— OUR ADVICE

Are you four weeks postnatal or four years postnatal? It doesn't really matter. After having a baby you will always be officially "postnatal". Let's concentrate on the positives instead of feeling guilty or sad about your jelly belly – let's remember why it's like that: your body has just done something amazing, it has made another human, or even multiple humans. If you think of other vessels that grew things inside them (egg shells and pea pods) they are completely destroyed afterwards – so what's a few stretch marks and an extra little layer of cuddle?

To come away from this process unscathed would be impossible, and who wants that anyway? The changes to your body are reminders of how strong and selfless you have been, and a bit of saggy skin and some stretch marks are like your badges of honour!

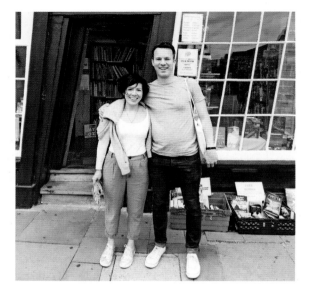

About sex after a baby

Clio Wood @andbreathewellbeing
andbreathewellbeing.com

Nobody tells you how much sex might hurt. About how it might damage me and my husband emotionally. About how it might feel like shards of glass cutting my vagina. About how long it would take me to rehabilitate physically and about how long it would take my marriage to recover.

    With a three-day labour, traumatic birth that included forceps and an episiotomy, postnatal depression and hypertonic (too tight) pelvic floor that took a year to be diagnosed, sex wasn't a walk in the park. My husband was understanding and didn't push it in the slightest, but I like to be in control and I hated myself for not living up to my perceived societal standards.

I was pushed from GP, to gynaecologist, to internal ultrasound and back again without a diagnosis or help. Nobody told me that perhaps a women's health physiotherapist was the answer. I had to find it out myself, over 12 months into my postnatal journey.

I had hypersensitive scarring, emotional barriers, identity issues, and super-tight muscles that bore witness to the understandable tension I felt after becoming a mother, but there was no information to guide or reassure me, no one to point me in the right direction. Once I found the right path, my recovery was long but straight-forward. I'm grateful and overjoyed that our sex life, communication and relationship are now better than ever. Nobody told me I could ever hope for that either.

——— OUR ADVICE

Having sex after having a baby will depend very much on your birth experience, how you have recovered, mentally and physically, and also, surprisingly, the way in which you are feeding your baby.

Most couples have had sex by about six to eight weeks. Many report having sex before their 6-week check as they have heard that the GP will ask about this.

Many women say that sex is just as enjoyable as it was before they had a baby. Some find that it is even better. But others may find it uncomfortable and even painful. If you experience pain or discomfort then please do go and speak to your GP about it and ask them to refer you to a gynaecologist or women's health physiotherapist. If for some reason you do not want to talk to your GP about this, you can make yourself a private appointment with a gynaecologist or women's health physiotherapist and they will be able to offer you some help.

Let's talk about sex . . .

—— DID YOU KNOW THAT THE WAY YOU FEED YOUR BABY CAN AFFECT YOUR SEX DRIVE?

Very often, the way you're feeding your baby has a bigger impact on your sex life than whether or not your baby came out of your vagina! Breastfeeding mothers have low levels of oestrogen and testosterone and high levels of prolactin which combine to depress your libido and make your vagina dry and uncomfortable during sex.

—— YOU MAY JUST NOT BE "UP FOR IT"

New mothers also complain of feeling "touched out". If they spend all day holding a baby or being grabbed and poked in the boobs, and covered in their own or their baby's bodily fluids then quite often they just do not want to be touched any more by anyone else. That feeling, combined with the complete exhaustion that comes with a new baby, can mean sex may be bottom of the agenda for a while!

Try to talk to your partner about this and explain how you're feeling, and try and think of some other things you can do to maintain your closeness until you are ready to have sex again.

However, if you do want to have sex, then there is no reason why you cannot, as long as everything has healed, but you might need to use some lubricant to make it a more comfortable and enjoyable experience.

—— DON'T FORGET ABOUT CONTRACEPTION!

If you do not want to conceive, you should use some form of contraception. Breastfeeding is not a fool-proof method of contraception. If you wish to take the contraceptive pill while you are breastfeeding then your doctor can prescribe you the mini-pill which will not cross over into your breast milk.

What's the best advice?

– Part 1 –

We asked our amazing community at @**amotherplace**
to share the best advice they received:

Pull up the drawbridge

Build your tribe

Don't be afraid to ask for help

It's ok not to be on your A game constantly –
the laundry and dirty pans can wait

Get your visitors to bring food. Baby never
goes hungry but mums do!

Warm baths to soothe sore bits and arnica
tablets for bruising

Take each day as it comes, don't rush to get
out of the house

Baby blues are normal, don't be embarrassed

Stay in bed and enjoy being waited on

There is no such thing as giving a baby too many cuddles

Drink lots of water

Don't be afraid to talk about how you're feeling
– dads too!

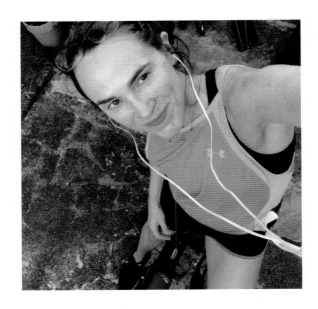

Incontinence is common but not normal

Jane Wake @janewakeuk

janewake.com

My firstborn came out very quickly – with his hand up like Superman! Being a sporty, I-can-do-anything, tough girl, I just thought all was fine and I could resume normal activities soon. Normal activity for me included running – not just as a hobby, it was my job as an official coach for the London Marathon.

About six months postnatal, I went out for a long run and I got caught short, I mean really short! Crossing my legs wasn't gonna cut it and I had to limp home with more than my tail between my legs!

That's how I found out about bladder and bowel incontinence.

A camera up the bum revealed I had an internal tear but that it would heal. I went to see a women's health physiotherapist. They are wonderful people who can internally examine you to check all your muscles and organs are doing what they should be. Often problems don't seem apparent at first, or we laugh them off: "Oops, I peed myself again!" Sometimes it only happens when you start to exercise more or perhaps even much later in life when your hormones start to change. While all of this is VERY common, none of it is normal and we shouldn't have to live with it. So go seek help AND DO YOUR PELVIC FLOOR EXERCISES! I am no longer a marathon trainer but a pelvic floor exercise specialist.

——— OUR ADVICE

Stress incontinence is common after a baby, but it isn't normal. You should not just accept this as something you have to live with for the rest of your life. There is a lot of help out there, but you can start by trying to help yourself at home with pelvic floor exercises which can help to prevent and also treat some cases of incontinence.

Pelvic floor exercises are designed to strengthen the muscles around the vagina, bladder and back passage. If you exercise yours regularly then you are less likely to suffer from incontinence after having a baby. We have some great tips on pages 38–41).

If you find that pelvic floor exercises are not helping, then please see your GP who can refer you to a women's health physiotherapist. The waiting lists are usually long, so some women prefer to see one privately. You may only need one session with a good physio. It is a very intimate appointment, so don't be shocked when you get an internal examination. It should be completely comfortable and you don't need to be embarrassed.

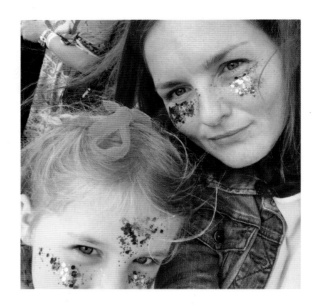

Your hair might fall out!

Hattie Mauleverer @hattiemauleverer
hattiemauleverer.co.uk

I have always had thickish wavy-ish hair that I can't grow below my shoulders. I don't do anything to it, cut it twice a year only. When I was pregnant I didn't really notice it being thicker or glossier, I got the general comments of how glowing I looked, but I was eating super well and not drinking!

Now I have my miracle four-month-old. Everywhere I look I see strands of my hair. I clean my hairbrush daily, clog the shower frequently. After my daughter, now four, I lost my hair too. Not clumps, but it might as well have been. I was distraught. My stretch marks didn't cause me as much anguish, they could be covered up. But my hair!

I sent my husband to get a special expensive hairbrush, got special shampoo, had a haircut, but still I moulted. For me it was one of the worst things postpartum. Everything else was manageable. Having gone through that with my first child, I know now that I only have a few more months till I am back to normal hair. But the loss of it daily still freaks me out!

—— OUR ADVICE

Hair loss after having a baby is completely normal so please don't worry. When you are pregnant your body produces more oestrogen, which makes your hair grow, which explains why loads of women report having amazing hair when they're pregnant. After you have had your baby and your oestrogen levels start to return to normal, you can guess what happens. But don't worry, you will not end up bald, your head is just shedding some of the extra hair it grew during your pregnancy. The loss will start to slow down and after a while your hair-growing cycles will get back to normal. You may notice hair loss more around the front of your hair, and this can be a real pain as it looks tufty when it starts to grow back. It can be a great excuse for a new haircut and some well-deserved me-time!

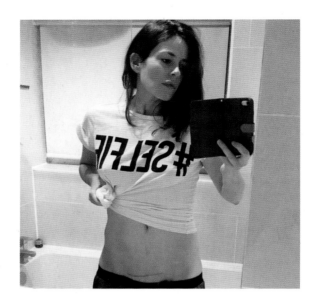

You may just love your scar

Ellie Thompson @jelliediary

Here is my six-month caesarean scar in all its glory. It feels quite rigid now, a bit like a thin piece of string. I was so squeamish about it for the first couple of months or so. It itches if I forget to apply cream once a day, and it is slightly sore when it's bashed in any way, but only momentarily. I'm not going to lie, I'm weirdly fond of it, because girls can rock scars too! AND it goes without saying that I'm proud of it too. I never thought I would be able to be a mum; for me, it's a reminder that my body isn't as useless as I had felt it was for so long. A scar is a journey or a story that got you to where you are today, and this beauty is definitely considered a lucky one.

—— OUR ADVICE

A scar can be a reminder of an important episode in your life, and what is more amazing than a scar which represents new life? Did you know that C-section scars are slightly curved and sometimes look like a little smile?

Make sure you take good care of your scar in the days and weeks after your C-section. Keep an eye on how it looks and feels and if it gets more sore, red or hot to the touch then you should speak to your GP as soon as you can, as those can be signs of infection.

Fresh scars can look quite alarming and many women do not want to look at theirs as it makes them feel squeamish. But your scar should be low down and in your pubic hair. It will fade as the years go on and there will be a time when you forget you have it.

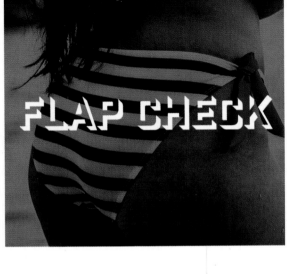

There may be some permanent changes

Anon

I gave birth to my first child naturally and without pain relief, but immediately afterwards I was whisked off to theatre to have an epidural and extensive stitches because I had torn badly inside and out.

I wasn't too bothered as I was preoccupied with my gorgeous new baby boy, and as I wasn't considering pursuing a career in porn! The thought of what my bits looked like was far from my mind and, the prevailing effects of sleep deprivation meant that I had no intention of ever having sex again. So who cared, right?! WRONG!

We had sex eventually, about nine months after I'd given birth, but even then it was traumatic. I was so worried that I looked ugly down south and I did not want my husband to see or feel this. I couldn't relax and the experience was really painful.

My labia were saggy and stretched beyond recognition. Even now, six years on with two kids, I am very self-conscious about it. Intimacy is still terrifying and when I wear a bikini, I panic that something is hanging out!

I don't want to have any more children, but I would like to be intimate with my husband again without feeling disgusting "down there" or worrying about what he thinks.

—— OUR ADVICE

Your vagina and vulva will feel and look different if you have a vaginal birth. Usually, things heal very quickly and although it may never look exactly how it did pre-pregnancy, it will get less sore and start to look better over the next few weeks.

Some women will experience a more significant physical change to their vulva and this can be upsetting and embarrassing to experience. It's an awkward thing for many women to talk about, but it is important to know that you are not alone and that plenty of women have similar symptoms and experiences after having a baby. If you are particularly worried you can speak to your midwife or GP about this and they may be able to refer you to a specialist.

You may find that confiding in your partner or a friend makes you feel better. Please do not suffer alone thinking you're the only one going through this, because you're not.

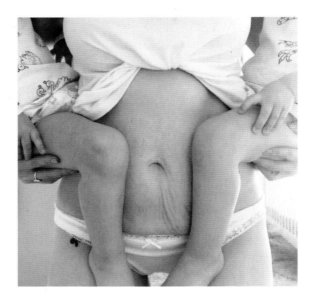

How to "bounce back"

Trudi Eade @trudi_eade

Almost every day, I receive messages from other mums asking me how I look the way that I do. How I got my "pre-baby body" back. Here's the truth, ladies – I DIDN'T. I have the excess skin. I don't have stomach definition the way I used to. My hips are a little wider. I don't want there to be any misconceptions. My body did not just "bounce back".

Now having said that, I work very hard to maintain a healthy lifestyle and to FEEL good in my skin. I may not ever look the way I did before I had the twins. And you know what? I'm ok with that. I have arms. I have legs. I can see, hear and experience life. My body has done amazing things, why on earth would I punish it?

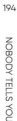

Learn to appreciate what you have. It doesn't mean you have to stop working for what you want, just show a little self-love along the way.

—— OUR ADVICE
Some of us are blessed with genes that will have us back in our skinny jeans hours after giving birth. Some of us are likely to hold on to a few kilos for a few months while hormones rise and fall and milk comes in and then goes, returning to work looking like nothing happened. Some of us will hold on to the softness for a little longer, maybe forever. The lucky ones will be happy with their new round edges, new role in life and new wardrobe, while some will lament this change in their shape daily. They will beat themselves up over the muffin tops that spill over their jeans or the hint of an extra chin. For some of us, the muffin top is related to actual muffin consumption, and for some it's a genetically predetermined disposition.

It's all normal. It's all ok. Things will change when you have a baby, physically and psychologically; no one becomes a mother without your body or soul changing in some way. It's just not possible, so be kind to yourself.

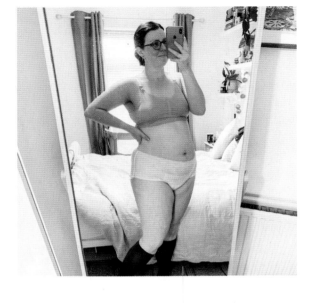

About recovering from a caesarean

Kim Lawler @finestimaginary

Nappies and compression socks are my new wardrobe staples! Here I am 50 hours after my baby boy was C-sectioned out. I'm battered and bruised, covered with needle holes from various tests and injections, and with a significant scar-to-be just above my pubes. Hello new body! My bump has pretty much gone already, there's some swelling from the C-section and my tummy's soft while everything knots itself back together. My boobs have started to get bigger now that my milk's on its way, and my nipples are already sore from our first forays into breastfeeding.

I'm so proud of my body, for growing a human, trying to push him out for a bit, dealing with major surgery and then being able to feed the little lad once he was safely here. Before, a C-section was my worst nightmare, now it's a crowning achievement. We didn't have the "conventional"/natural birth that I'd hoped for in any way, shape or form, but the outcome was still the same, just with a different healing process.

———— OUR ADVICE

After a caesarean section, the first four to six hours of care will be in the high-dependency area to look out for complications such as bleeding. Your catheter and intravenous drip will be removed after 12 to 24 hours. You may have a drain to remove fluid from the abdomen, which will also be removed after 24 hours. Stitches will usually be removed after four or five days or if they are dissolvable then they will not need removing. A feeling of numbness around the scar is normal, and this will usually wear off over the following weeks.

You will usually lose blood from the placental site, through your vagina, in the same way as a woman who has had a vaginal birth. You will probably also experience the same after-pains as your uterus contracts after the birth. You may also experience pain from the wound and also from abdominal wind. Our advice is to say "yes" to all the drugs you are offered for pain relief for the first 24 to 48 hours, and then take them as required. They are designed to make you feel comfortable while you heal and they are safe for breastfeeding.

You may feel pain or discomfort when you reach to pick up your baby, so just take it slowly and get someone to help you the first few days.

The average length of stay in hospital is three days and usually by day 5 you will be feeling much better.

CONTENTS

Feeding your baby

Breastfeeding is a wonderful way of nourishing your baby and some women are lucky enough to take to it easily and enjoy it. Many others struggle for a multitude of reasons and it is important to offer support for all who need it. Breast is best in many circumstances, but it's important that we acknowledge that it's not always possible. There is no shame in formula-feeding your baby and you deserve to feed however you need to without fear of judgement.

This chapter is dedicated to stories from mums who have fed by bottle and/or breast and are doing the best for their families. Alongside our advice, their stories will fill you in on all the things that Nobody Tells You . . .

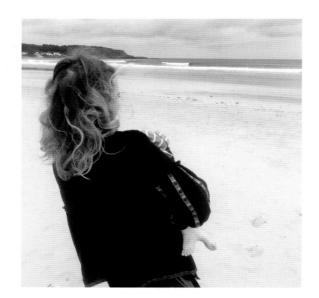

Breastfeeding can be a joy!

Gemma Brown @gemmaruthbrown
gemmaruthbrown.com

It was something I knew I wanted to try, but honestly? I was terrified! I'd heard so much about tongue tie, latch and supply issues, allergies etc. that I didn't realise what a JOY breastfeeding could be.

It was difficult to begin with: his blood sugars were tested regularly so I felt under pressure to get feeding sorted, while not having a clue what I was doing! I remember 11pm on our first night . . . two midwives trying to squeeze microscopic droplets of colostrum out of my boob while my husband looked on in shock. I found hospital support confusing. But I met one midwife who, after giving me some basic tips, simply had the confidence in me that

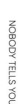

I needed in order to have confidence in myself. She just said, "You're going to do this." And I did.

We dealt with slow weight gain and jaundice at the beginning as well as mastitis and thrush later on, but me and my silver nipple cups powered on through and here we are, 18 months later and still going strong.

Breastfeeding is an essential tool in my mothering kit. It is still Baby B's "safe place" – so it's what we do when he bumps his head or grazes his knee, when he's feeling tired or unsure, when he's a little chilly in winter or in the heat of summer, when he just needs a little comfort or down time. It's also a super-quick way to get him back to sleep during those nightly wakes!

And now that I'm back to work, it's a lovely way to enjoy a quiet moment together before I leave, and to connect when I come back. Breastfeeding is one of the best things I have ever done. I love it!

—— OUR ADVICE

This is brilliant to hear. While there are lots of women who struggle with breastfeeding, there are also many women who have a really wonderful experience. Some mothers and their babies just take to it straight away and find the whole thing easy and enjoyable. Some find it hard at the start but it can often get much more comfortable and easier with expert advice and the passage of time.

We all know that under most circumstances, breast is best, we don't need anyone to remind us about that, so even if you are feeling nervous about breastfeeding, we would encourage you to give it your best shot and you never know, you may just love it. And if you don't, that's ok, too.

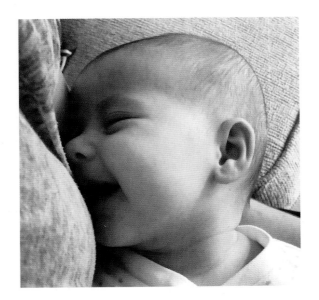

You might struggle to breastfeed

Ashley White @ashleyclairwhite

Nobody tells you that even if your baby has the perfect latch, you might still have difficulties with breastfeeding. Nobody told me no matter how open-minded you wanted to be, how sad you would feel when it didn't quite work out. Nobody told me the endless hours of cluster feeding could make you feel like your body wasn't providing for your baby like it's supposed to. Nobody told me how inferior you could feel bottle-feeding your baby in a room full of breastfeeding mothers. Nobody told me when your milk begins to dry up, you feel like a little part of you is missing. Nobody told me how heartbreakingly hard the decision to stop would be.

I wish I had found more support while I was pregnant; I would have felt so much better equipped for what was in store for us. I wish I had been given more realistic information on what a breastfeeding journey could look like. I wish I could turn back the clock and try again.

—— OUR ADVICE

Many women struggle to breastfeed for a variety of reasons and often do not manage to find the support they need to deal with these problems and continue to breastfeed. Giving up breastfeeding at any time can cause women to feel very upset and low for a few days. This is often explained by the huge hormone change as oxytocin and prolactin levels drop when your milk starts to dry up. But for women who feel that they were forced to give up feeding because of factors beyond their control, such as pain, infection, illness, social or professional issues, the feelings of guilt and shame can last much longer.

But please don't feel guilty. You've probably heard it a million times, but a happy and healthy mother is important for a happy baby. As long as your baby is being fed and is also happy and healthy then sometimes that is the very best we can do.

There is a lot of pressure put upon women to be able to breastfeed, but we are not often equipped with all the facts and enough support to make this possible. We all know the mantra "breast is best" but it is important to understand that if you need to give your baby formula, this is not a failure on your part. In a few years' time, you will be standing in a playground and you will not be able to tell the breastfed toddlers from the bottle-fed ones . . . they will all be eating dirt and running around like red-faced loons!

On co-sleeping

I am in my happy place
Hopefully I'll be asleep soon
But while I'm awake
This moment I will take
To savour this perfection
That is you two

My boobs feel empty
But that's okay
My girls and my bed are full

One snores softly down by my feet
the other farts a tune into the sheets

And that is all it takes
For me to feel great
For me to feel grateful

Chaneen Saliee @chaneensaliee

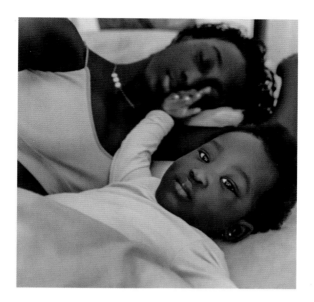

About co-sleeping

Chaneen Saliee @chaneensaliee
chicanddiscreet.com

I wish someone told me that co-sleeping feels so good, so natural and so instinctive. I tried to put my babies to sleep in their cot but it didn't feel right. Having them in bed with me makes us all feel safe and close.

    Now they are older I am trying to get them to sleep by themselves, but they creep back to my bed again in the night. There is no rush, I guess. If they feel more secure with me, then that's ok.

───── OUR ADVICE

Bed-sharing or co-sleeping is an ancient, worldwide cultural practice that is still popular especially with breastfeeding mothers. But more recently parents have been alerted to the potential risks associated with co-sleeping, namely an increase in the likelihood of SIDS (Sudden Infant Death Syndrome).

Advice about co-sleeping varies from country to country, depending on breastfeeding rates and also the most recent research. The results of studies done on the safety of co-sleeping can often seem confusing and contradictory so it is really important that people have access to enough information to make an informed choice.

In the UK, parents are encouraged to look at the risks and benefits of co-sleeping, based on their own individual circumstances, and to make a decision that feels safe for them. You can find out more information about safer sleeping from The Lullaby Trust.

What's the best advice?

– Part 2 –

We asked our amazing community at **@amotherplace**
to share the best advice they received:

Give visitors a job when they come over

Ban visitors unless they are useful

Stop trying to do everything

A walk around the block can save your sanity

Nobody knows what they're doing straight away

Have a basket of supplies by the sofa –
changing stuff, chocolate, remote control

Get some nice PJs so you can feel half decent for
visitors without having to get properly dressed

Everything is a phase

Tomorrow is a new day

You need to be able to look after yourself to look
after baby

Trust your instincts

If baby is fed/winded/clean/warm and still crying
it's ok to pop them in a basket/cot and have a shower

A routine can save your sanity

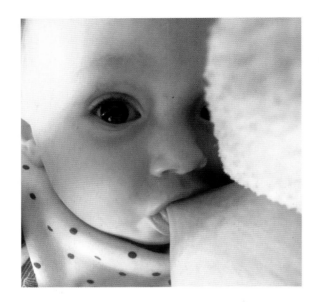

About cluster feeding

Chloe Milne @chloebythecoast

Before I had a baby I knew about sore nipples and leaky boobs. I even knew about tongue tie and mastitis. But nobody explained that some days a newborn does almost nothing but eat. Nobody warned me that sometimes I'd sit down for a feed at 5pm and we'd still be going in the early hours of the morning. Nobody had uttered the words "cluster feeding" to me, or had thought to mention growth spurts and how it was totally normal to be stuck under a ravenous baby for hours and hours and hours and . . . hours.

Cluster feeding is like a marathon in not moving. It involves putting a lot of time into sitting comfortably while feeding a baby who seems impossible to fill. It doesn't sound so tough now that I write it down, but it's hard going. The relentlessness of it will wear you down and you'll feel like you want to give up. But you can do it. Know that cluster feeding is completely normal, and you will get through it. Give in to it, get the telly on, have people bring you whatever you need, and enjoy the time just sitting. Looking back, I wish I'd embraced those long shifts on the sofa more.

Breastfeeding's not for everyone, but if it is for you and you're yet to embark on the journey, know that your couch is going to be right there with you. Go with the cluster feeds and enjoy the beauty that is keeping your baby alive with nothing but your boobs – you are a superwoman!

—— OUR ADVICE

Cluster feeding is when babies space feeding closer together at certain times of the day, usually the evening. It is very common but it can be frustrating and exhausting for new mums. There is not much you can do about it except make sure you are comfortable and have everything you need close to hand. Make sure you have lots of water, lots of biscuits and that the remote control/phone/book is within reach!

Pretty soon when your baby starts crawling, there won't be much time for sitting on the sofa, so try and relax and remember that, and enjoy just being with your baby.

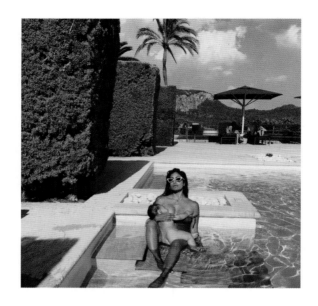

How to prepare for breastfeeding in public

Shayoon Mendeluk @shayoon_

I've been travelling a lot this summer, and unfortunately many places, especially in the UK and the United States, frowned upon public breastfeeding! I was asked to leave or move to the bathroom at not one but three different restaurants! A restaurant, an establishment where you go to eat. Ironically they felt it was shameful to feed my newborn publicly.

There is absolutely nothing wrong with breastfeeding your child in public. To me, it is the most beautiful, primal and natural thing to do. I come from a culture where shame . . . coverage . . . hiding . . . is engrained into our children and women. I grew up Muslim, I grew up in Indian and Pakistani culture. I grew up conditioned and programmed to think that I need to feel some sort of shame for showing my body. Today I would like to say shame on you if you project any sort of negativity to a mother that is feeding her child, no matter her colour, no matter her race, no matter her religion. Instead, praise women for their sacrifice in bringing these beautiful blessings to this earth.

—— OUR ADVICE

It can be nerve-wracking to breastfeed in public for the first time. You get braver the more times you do it and you learn that people are busy and consumed with their own business and hardly spare you a glance unless they disapprove (idiots) or are perverts (also idiots). And don't worry about any perverts, as you get so fast at whipping down your top and latching the baby on that there is nothing for even the beadiest-eyed wrong'un to see! As for the disapprovers, well hopefully you won't run into any of those, but if you do, hold your head high and try and ignore them. In the UK you are entitled to breastfeed in public at any time and in any place. It is illegal for anyone to ask a breastfeeding woman to leave a public place, such as a cafe, shop or public transport.

If you feel nervous, it can be a good idea to take a friend with you the first time you feed in public. Wear clothing and a bra that make breastfeeding easier so you don't have to start getting undressed. You can use a large scarf or muslin if you want to try and cover yourself up when you feed, although some mums find that this can attract even more unwanted attention. Take a deep breath and just do it and you will be fine!

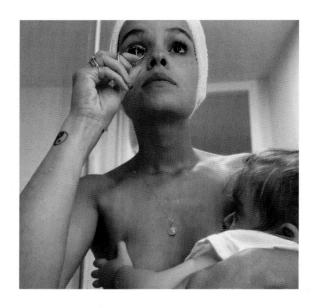

We should be honest about feeding

Maria Betsworth @milkmakingmama
milkmakingmama.co.uk

Nobody tells you how time-consuming breastfeeding can really be. Nobody is transparent about what breastfeeding is really like, the ups and downs, the emotions involved every day, the commitment and struggles. Why is that? Are we afraid to admit what we are feeling or do we not want to scare others off? Motherhood is a challenge on a daily basis. Breastfeeding, pumping, bottle-feeding all come with ups and downs but the real picture of what it is truly like is hidden behind closed doors. Nobody tells you the physical and mental exhaustion you can feel from being sleep deprived but having to function each day. Nobody tells you that you will have very little time on your own, nobody tells you that your body now belongs to your babies, taking from you what they need. But you will gladly give.

I will give the last minute of my sleep, the last drop of milk, I will pump for 365 days, and I will breastfeed until you are ready to stop, I will give in to your every need, and I will learn to become the mama you need me to be.

It is ok to admit that this motherhood thing is hard. It is more than ok to dislike certain aspects of mothering yet still want to be a mama. Let's help each other with the reality of what things are going to be like and support each other along this journey of motherhood, without judgement of how each of us is mothering or what tools we are using to feed; breast or bottle, in the end all that matters is a happy, cared-for and loved baby.

—— OUR ADVICE

Yes we must be honest, for the sake of those new parents coming behind us. It's not fair for us to shroud the realities of parenthood in secrecy. If someone asks your opinion on any aspect of pregnancy, birth or motherhood, then we think that being honest about the good and the bad bits is the right thing.

So many parts of parenting are wonderful and rewarding, and other parts feel tough and relentless. If we know this in advance then perhaps this will help us to prepare for these tricky times. Breastfeeding is not always a doddle, and we must be realistic about this and set ourselves up with realistic expectations.

If you are experiencing a difficult time, it can help to remember that "everything is a phase". The sore nipples and sleepless nights will not last forever, so do not despair.

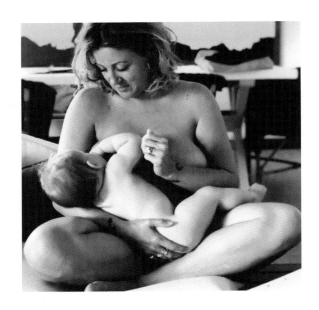

Giving up breastfeeding can feel emotional

Clemmie Telford @clemmie_telford
motherofalllists.com

Nobody tells you how it feels when you stop breastfeeding.
I've decided to wean Greta from the boob. I didn't have any
preconceived ideas of how long we'd go on for. I always hoped it'd
become obvious when the right time to stop was. And I believe it's
now. I'm finding it increasingly draining and less rewarding. It's been
such a wonderful experience that I want to leave on a positive. We
went out with a bang too: with a boob in the bath, just the two of us.
Gahhhhh, parenting is emotional! My husband Ben keeps

catching me sobbing about it – even though I know it's the right decision, it's the end of a very special chapter. Time to reclaim "the girls" as mine after a sterling effort of 33 months nursing my three babes.

—— OUR ADVICE

Nobody tells you when to stop breastfeeding. There isn't often an exact time when you decide "Right, that's it". It's usually a decision that comes on slowly and is based upon practical and emotional considerations.

- sometimes it can feel selfish (even though it isn't)
- sometimes it can feel necessary
- sometimes it can feel premature or forced
- sometimes it can feel devastating
- sometimes it can feel like a huge relief
- sometimes we stop feeding because it's too painful/ difficult/time-consuming/impractical to carry on
- sometimes we have to stop feeding to go back to work

Whatever your reason for stopping, your oxytocin and prolactin levels will drop dramatically, which in itself can make you feel very emotional as your milk starts to dry up. Don't worry about feeling teary for a few days. This is very common and usually only temporary. If you experience longer-lasting emotional issues after stopping breastfeeding, please talk to your GP.

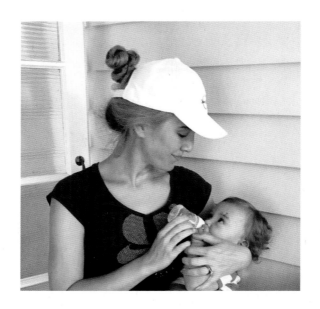

You may feel judged for bottle-feeding

Lisa Schmidt @lisaschmidt84

Nobody tells you about the stigma attached to bottle-feeding. I would love to help end this. How often do you see images of women bottle-feeding their babies? It's very rare. It's unfortunate that society has made women feel ashamed of feeding their babies in this manner. There could be numerous reasons why someone chooses to bottle-feed and what I dislike most is the judgement cast and the looking down at your decision for whatever reason that may be.

I'm such a believer in positivity. Let's support one another. We all know the famous saying "fed is best" and that's all there really is to it. I have so much support and admiration for breastfeeding mamas too and I know they face their own challenges from the public.

—— OUR ADVICE

Many women report feeling judged for their decision to bottle/formula-feed. This is very sad because there are just so many different reasons, ranging from medical to social issues, that may explain why someone might have chosen to bottle-feed, so it is not for others to pass judgement on this.

There are circumstances where bottle/formula-feeding may actually be the best thing for the baby and these are often complicated and personal. You know your reasons for bottle-feeding your baby and it will not be a decision that was made lightly, so stick to your guns and try not to worry about what others think, as you know you're doing the best for your baby and that is what's important.

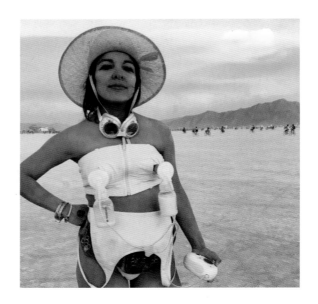

About expressing milk

Miki Agrawal @mikiagrawal
mikiagrawal.com

A month after Hiro's birth, I decided that it was time to pump extra milk in preparation for my three-night trip to Burning Man a month later to surprise my twin sister because her boyfriend was going to propose to her. I calculated that Hiro needed about 32 bags of milk (eight per day) to go and so I started pumping one or two extra bags of milk per day for the month prior and diligently dated all of the bags and put them in the freezer in chronological order of when I pumped. It was wild to see a freezer full of MY harvest of MY body – I mean come on, insane right?!

I used an electric pump and I think this is where my rock-hard-painful-boobs era began. My boobs would pump so much extra milk that they ballooned and became so hard and I remember having to wake Hiro up a few times to let him bring them down (luckily he did very quickly).

At Burning Man, I realised that I had to keep expressing because the milk wouldn't just stop, it would keep coming and I wanted to make sure that Hiro was still breastfeeding when I got back so I had to pump and pump while I was there. I did not want to waste my breast milk so I gave it out for people to drink, and make lattes and White Russians with!

—— OUR ADVICE

There are lots of reasons why you might want to try expressing milk. It is so handy if you want someone else to feed your baby because you have to be apart from them for a while, or if you just want a break from feeding and you have a willing and able volunteer.

Some new mums get stressed trying to pump, to create a store of milk for their freezer. They like the idea of a partner doing a night feed, so spend ages trying to save a feed's worth of milk for their stash. But the reality is, this can be very difficult when you are still establishing breastfeeding. Your body will be very responsive to the amount of milk you take from it and the more you take, the hungrier it thinks your baby is and so produces more and more milk. If you are not removing this milk by pumping or feeding then your breasts can quickly become engorged and sore.

So take it easy and start slowly, don't go into pumping overdrive. If you are very keen to have back-up milk then ensure you pump roughly the same amount every day so that your milk supply knows what to expect.

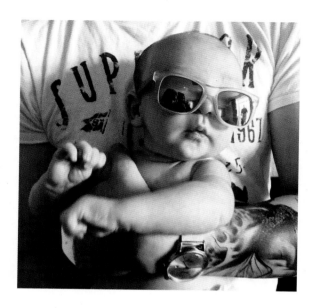

Tongue tie can be a big deal

Tilly Barfield-Jones @tillybar_jones

Pretty much as soon as our son Ollie let out his first cry, one of the midwives spotted that he had "a bit of tongue tie". It was very much downplayed in hospital. We were told it could cause problems feeding, and possibly speech problems later in life, but that it was optional for us to have it treated as it was more than likely it would cause no problems at all.

Over the next couple of days I really struggled to feed Ollie, as it became more and more painful for me and more and more stressful for him. He was chewing my nipples and he couldn't get enough milk to satisfy his hunger. We were put in touch with a private clinician to treat his tongue tie, as getting referred through the NHS can be tricky and long-winded.

Once we contacted the private lactation consultant, we were seen the next day and she instantly spotted that "a bit of tongue tie" was actually quite severe. He couldn't get his tongue past his teeth at all. No wonder he couldn't feed!

After explaining the procedure and healing process, the consultant swaddled Ollie so he couldn't wriggle and snipped the tight bit of skin under his tongue. He let out a short yelp but didn't cry, and that was it! It was a simple procedure which caused minimal fuss and he was able to feed much better.

—— OUR ADVICE

Tongue tie is a tricky one. It is not checked for or dealt with routinely in the UK at the moment and this is because plenty of babies can feed very successfully with a tongue tie and so the NHS deems it unnecessary to offer a procedure unless there are actually feeding problems. This is understandable, but it can lead to distressing situations where babies do not feed well and referrals for getting the tie snipped can take longer than we would like. It is possible to get this done privately, and you may be able to get some details about this from your midwife or GP.

The procedure is not the most pleasant thing to experience but please don't worry as it is not particularly distressing for your baby and they are usually very happy to be able to feed more effectively immediately afterwards.

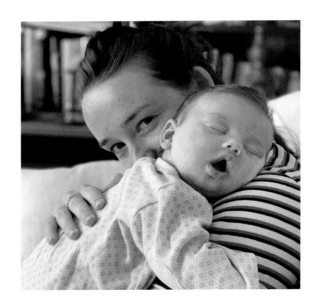

About choosing not to breastfeed

Charlotte Parsley

Pre-pregnancy I hadn't thought much about how I might feed my own baby. As a midwife, I suppose I'd always assumed I would breastfeed.

When I fell pregnant, I suffered from hyperemesis gravidarum and spent 36 weeks vomiting, taking medication and counting down the days to labour.

This little person had taken over my body and my mind from the start and I didn't feel like me any more.

I wanted to feel sexy. I did not want to smell of sour milk.

I did not want to leak through my tops. I wanted feeding to be a bonding experience, not riddled with stress and anxiety. My husband wanted to help. I wanted to protect my mental health. I wanted to have a gin and tonic!

I never got the overwhelming maternal urge to breastfeed; I saw it as a means to feed her, for me it wasn't enjoyable and I spent each feed counting down the minutes. If someone had asked me how I felt, I would have said I was indifferent to it.

I reflect on our journey with a little sadness – if I had had an easier pregnancy maybe I would have continued to breastfeed.

Each feeding journey is so personal, but I don't have any regrets because for us, this works and we're both happy and healthy.

—— OUR ADVICE

There are many different psychological and physical reasons why breastfeeding may not work out for some mums and babies. We all know that breastfeeding provides many recognised benefits, but life is not always that simple or easy for everyone. We are lucky that we live in a world where we have choices and alternatives and if for some reason you cannot breastfeed your baby then there are a number of infant formulas you can use.

Please consider the financial implications of having to add formula to your shopping list, and consult a healthcare professional to help you make an informed choice before deciding not to breastfeed.

CONTENTS

You are
not alone

Being a parent is simultaneously wonderful and crappy, rewarding yet back-breaking and both smile- and tear-inducing all at the same time.

This last chapter is full of stories that tell it how it is and reassure you that however you're feeling, you are most definitely NOT alone.

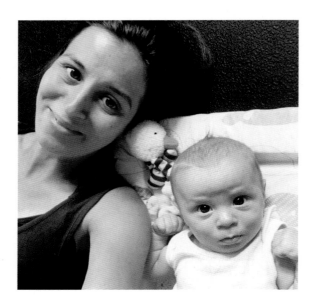

You will get so much unsolicited advice

Elizabeth Davies @themummycoach.co.uk
themummycoach.co.uk

Nobody tells you that, once you have a baby, everybody – from well-meaning relatives to the man behind the checkout in the supermarket – will have an opinion about how you are doing things. In fact, not just some "things", but everything.

"Oh you're burping your baby? No, no, no; you don't need to burp your baby, just let the wind come up naturally."

"You're not burping your baby? The poor thing. She'll never settle unless you burp her."

"That's not how I used to burp my babies when they were little. Try this way. And be sure to get some gripe water."

Looking back at that time, I don't think people were being deliberately mean or critical. It's just people get over-excited when there is a small baby around and, seemingly as a result, have to say something. Anything. When you are in a fog of sleep deprivation and hormones, though, and you're doing your very best to listen to your new baby's cries (because, apparently, she has a different cry for everything but, so far, they all sound the same to you) it can really undermine your confidence as a new parent.

——— OUR ADVICE

People who comment on your parenting methods, in general are well meaning and they don't mean to be irritating, but they damn well can be! It is so hard when you're trying to find your way, learning to trust your instincts and settle into this new role and people seem to be questioning your decisions and your methods.

If you don't want it to drive you bonkers, you'll have to learn to take a deep breath and just smile and say "thanks". And actually, try and keep an open mind, because for every dozen crap bits of unwanted advice, you will come across some gems that you will be thankful for!

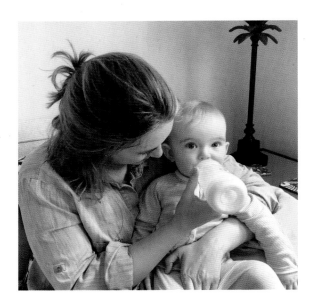

About colic and reflux

Katy Winskell @katywinskellrowe

Nobody told me that my baby wouldn't want to eat. I always knew breastfeeding might prove hard, or even impossible, but I never imagined that my baby wouldn't want to drink milk, from the breast or from the bottle. I had no idea that my maternity leave would often involve spending ten hours a day stuck at home trying to persuade my daughter to feed, while we both cried.

At first I thought my baby's reluctance to feed and the heartbreaking evenings of watching her scream for hours until she made herself sick must be colic. Nobody had told me about reflux.

It took several months for several clinicians to diagnose my daughter with severe silent reflux, and several more months to investigate the potential cause, which is looking like CMPA (Cows Milk Protein Allergy). She's sharp and made an association between the bottle and pain quickly, which meant getting her onto one of the foul-smelling prescription formulas was impossible and I'd packed in the pumping by then.

She's finally on a specialist formula that suits her, but I'm still apprehensive before every feed and weaning has been challenging. I adore her, but I wish I'd been better informed to know what to look for.

—— OUR ADVICE

Having a baby that doesn't feed well or one who is very uncomfortable after feeding is very stressful indeed and can really make life feel very hard in the postnatal period. Babies that are not feeding well for various reasons are often grouchy and this can affect their sleep. This affects mum too . . . and all around her!

Babies suffer from reflux when the muscle in their throat that is designed to keep food down is not yet properly developed. Milk can come back up again after they have finished feeding, which can cause a burning sensation and sometimes lead to vomiting.

SYMPTOMS OF REFLUX INCLUDE:
• vomiting after feeds (different to posseting which is just a small bit of milk coming back up)
• crying after feeds
• pulling away from feeds
• difficulty winding
• unexplained crying
• dislike of lying flat on back
• difficulty settling for naps

THINGS THAT MAY HELP A BABY WITH REFLUX:
• winding frequently throughout feeds
• feeding them in an upright position
• keeping them upright for a bit afterwards

If you think your baby is suffering from reflux then please speak to your GP or a qualified lactation consultant. You may have to push to get a referral from your GP as sometimes they do not have specialist knowledge of this condition in babies.

What's the worst advice?

We asked our amazing community at @**amotherplace** to share the worst advice they received. This is purely for entertainment so please don't take any of this advice seriously.

Don't hold her too much, you will make her bones soft

You should breastfeed your baby less often – you need to show her who's boss

Your three-month-old is manipulating you when she cries at night

Don't let him fall asleep while he is feeding

Give your baby Calpol every night

Make sure you enjoy every moment

Don't spoil your baby by holding him all the time

Don't use a sling as this will make a rod for your own back

You should think about shifting the baby weight

Stop worrying, all babies know how to breastfeed instinctively

Make sure you keep the house clean and give your husband sex or he will go elsewhere

Have your baby exorcised to get rid of eczema

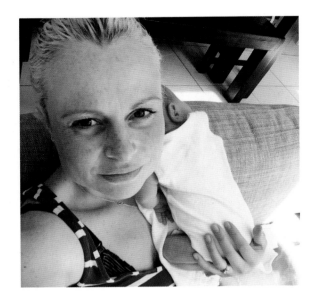

You might get the
bedtime dread

Sophie Constable @scbc79

Nobody tells you about the "bedtime dread" or "night fear". That your husband would look at you with pity at about 10.30pm and say, "Good luck". And you would feel sick because you didn't know how many times you would be woken by a hungry baby, or when. That it would be like you were about to sit an exam without having done any revision. Would you get 20 minutes? An hour? Two hours before the next feed? That feeling of dread watching the sun go down, knowing that it was going to be bad, you just didn't know how bad! And the feeling of relief and fear when at 3 or 4am you were sitting on WhatsApp feeding your baby and the sun started to come up. Knowing that the night was over but you were broken before the day had started.

—— OUR ADVICE

The fear is real! It's so tough going to bed knowing you're going to have a crap night's sleep and you're going to feel shit the next day. And even if you have the most supportive partner in the world, if you're breastfeeding, then most likely you will be up alone.

Clock-watching and counting the hours you have slept or not slept can be unhelpful and can even make you feel worse. If you're a certain personality type or a bit of a control freak then routine, sleep and feeding can become all-consuming and it's very hard to relax and be the chilled-out mum that you thought you might be.

No matter how many times people tell you that you will be tired, you just don't really get it until you're in it. But don't worry, it does get better . . . eventually!

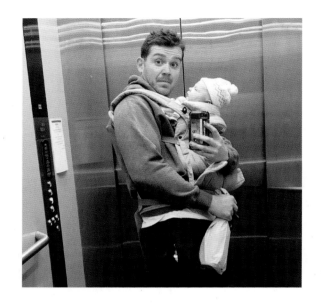

Babies cry when you put them down

Elizabeth Farrar @elizamacbeth_

Pre-baby, I used to make statements such as "babies won't die from crying" but I had no idea that the sound of her crying in the early days would absolutely rip my heart out and everything would be done quickly in between her tiny sleeps. Making myself presentable was important for me to feel put together, but it was a struggle most days. So, you actually cannot put your baby down for a good few weeks. Unless they are asleep, they demand to be in your arms (or back in your uterus).

Enjoy the cuddles of a newborn; soon they don't want to lie or sleep on you, and I miss that terribly! Nothing is more amazing than your baby sleeping on your chest; it doesn't last long and I didn't value it as much as I should have.

This picture is of my partner, who came home to give me a break and take our baby out to buy me wine, so I could drown my feelings of inadequacy and start the next day fresh. Every day is a new day.

———— OUR ADVICE

You pace the room with your baby until he falls still and silent in your arms . . . you decide to sit down on the sofa, or try and lie him in his cot . . . and . . . "WAAAAAAAAAAAAAAAAAAAAAAAAAAA!"

Well you're not alone, so don't worry. Apparently there are very good evolutionary reasons behind this. Basically, when we lived in caves and were in constant danger of being eaten by marauding beasts, a mother picking up her baby to flee from these predators would increase their chances of survival. By keeping quiet once she has done this, the baby would further increase these chances and apparently it is this instinct which still exists in babies today! So there you have some science to explain why your baby cries every time you put him down and stops when you pick him up. But this is not very helpful in those first few weeks and months when you just want to put your baby down so that you can have a shower.

There may be times when you have no option but to let your baby cry for a little bit while you shower and get dressed. It can feel very stressful, but your baby will not come to any harm if they cry for a few minutes while you wipe your bum or clean your teeth. As time goes on your baby will get used to not being in your arms all the time and will cry less and less when you put him down.

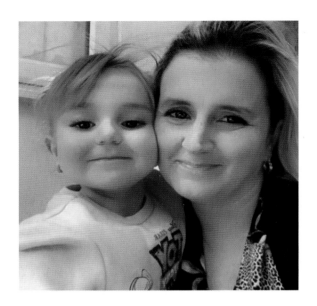

There is help out there if you need to go it alone

Victoria Jones

When I gave birth to my beautiful daughter I was so happy to finally become a mum and have a family of my own, but nobody told me how quickly my life was going to change.

Through my pregnancy I had doubts about my daughter's dad. He wasn't being honest with me and he became controlling and emotionally exhausted me with his lies. One day I spoke with my midwife about my money worries and the doubts I had been feeling about her dad. I was worried that if he left I would struggle with not having things for my daughter, so the midwife pointed me in the direction of Little Village, which is like a food bank but for baby equipment.

They were amazing and made an appointment for me to come in and get supplies for my daughter such as a cot, clothes, toys, books, nappies and wipes. They didn't just do that: they also gave me the strength to be the mum I wanted to be to my daughter. I was so stressed with her dad, my anxiety got worse and I felt like I had already failed her, but the volunteers I spoke to each time I went there gave me the strength to be me again.

My ex became very aggressive towards me and was increasingly negligent with our baby, so I stopped contact with him and had to seek advice from solicitors about what to do next. He threatened me, and I had no choice but to involve the police and go into hiding for about three weeks. After about a year of having advice and support from family and friends and especially Little Village, I felt strong enough to stand up and protect my baby girl, who is three now.

Little Village gave me everything I needed and the strength to be the mum my daughter needs. I felt low and weak but, thanks to them, I am stronger than ever. They gave me a part-time job in the crèche and I finally feel like I'm back to the person I was before I met him. Life is amazing and I love my daughter so much. I have family and Little Village to thank for that.

—— OUR ADVICE

Anyone can be a victim of domestic abuse, regardless of their age, ethnicity, socio-economic status or background. If you are living with a physically or psychologically abusive partner or you are worried about the safety of yourself or your children, then there is support available to you including police response, online help, phone lines and refuges.

There are charities and organisations that can help to get you to a safer place. They can help with housing, protecting you and your children, the legal side of things, the financials and psychological support to get you back on your feet.

It is so important that you understand that domestic abuse is never your fault and you do not have to live with it.

Little Village is a charity that collects great-quality donations of clothes, toys and kit for babies and children up to the age of five, and then gifts these donations on to local families who are dealing with really challenging circumstances – homelessness, unemployment, low wages and domestic violence. Families are sent their way by a network of referral partners – health visitors, children's centres and midwives primarily, but also faith organisations, other charities and public servants. Their dream is that no child grows up without essential items of clothing, toys and equipment. Find out more at @littlevillagehq or littlevillagehq.org.

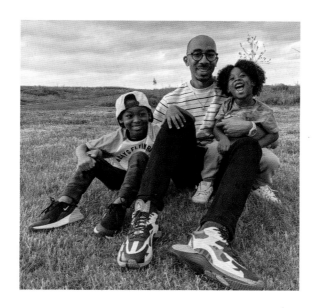

How to raise black children

Robert Douglas @this_father_life

Raising black children comes with all of the beautiful and exciting moments like raising any other child. However, parenting black children has a thick layer of racism to navigate and it's always present at the forefront of your minds. You not only have to think about how and when you talk to your children about racism and what lies ahead for them, but also simple things like hunting for books or TV programmes where they can see at least one person who looks like them, thinking about what damaging comments or attitudes they will face from children, teachers and

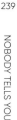

parents at school, or what box they will be forced into as they grow up.

I learned a lot from talking to parents of older black children and from my own father. It wasn't accessible via any parenting book or blog and we even had to do our own research to correct some healthcare professionals on health matters that impact black mothers and babies.

The phrase "you have to work twice as hard for half as much" is very real among the black community and, even if you don't verbalise it, you somehow find a way to demonstrate it to your children.

Our hopes and dreams for our children are the same as any other parent, but I know – no matter how hard they work, how skilled they are, how creative they are or how academic they become – there is an additional barrier they have to overcome that has nothing to do with how well they apply themselves. The reality of that barrier will hit them as it hit me.

Because of all this, there is a special kind of magic inside every black child. Seeing and discovering it is exciting.

—— OUR ADVICE

As parents, we want to keep our children safe, happy and healthy while instilling them with confidence and self-belief. The job is a tough and relentless one for all of us, but even more so for families who are faced with the daily struggle of overcoming racist preconceptions and barriers.

Even before your child is born, knowing that, as a black mother, you are five times more likely to die from complications during pregnancy and childbirth* is horrific. Then, starting life as a parent, realising your child will find life harder than their white peers is heartbreaking and downright unfair. Being aware that you will have to worry about your child more than white parents and that you will have to try to explain and rationalise things to your children that white people will never have to do is distressing and difficult to reconcile.

We have it within all of us to put an end to this inequality. We must advocate for all our fellow human beings, regardless of their race or skin colour. It is not good enough to just say you are not racist; if we are to overcome the inherent racism that black people face on a daily basis, we must all be actively anti-racist. We must speak up when we see or hear racism around us, at work, in public and – just as importantly – among friends and family at home.

* MBRRACE-UK Report 2018, 2019

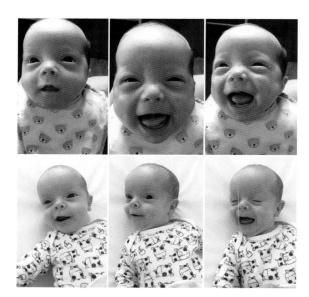

That first smile makes everything ok

Claire Muir @claire_roisin_freiya

When those first smiles appeared I truly accepted that all we had been through was worth it: the sudden early labour; the seven weeks of neonatal care; the chronic reflux; the endless hours sat expressing; the relentless feeding; the obscene lack of sleep; the fact our lives as we knew them and the people we were had virtually disappeared. I think before that we were in such a fug of mayhem and lack of sleep that we were just on autopilot struggling our way through the storm, and hadn't fully appreciated that we'd get through to the other side at some point.

Even at 15 months old all they have to do is smile and it totally dissolves a situation; I forget I'm mad because they won't eat the food I've spent time preparing; I forget I'm tired because I had one of them kicking me in the ribs all night; I forget I'm stressing about the housework I need to do or I forgot to get dinner out of the freezer; I forget I haven't got to drink wine with my best friends for months.

I like to think other people feel the same, that there are people out there who have had worse struggles than us who will soon see their newborns smile for the first time and it'll act like a medicine for their battle-scarred souls after all they've been through to reach that point.

—— OUR ADVICE

It's so true! A simple smile from your baby makes it all worth it. Babies usually smile between six and 12 weeks, and we think it's no coincidence that this is when you will probably be at your most tired and feeling completely overwhelmed. You've forgotten what a full night's sleep feels like, your days have become a blur of nappy changing and feeding and you may start to wonder if you're really cut out to be a parent after all . . . and then they smile!

It's amazing!

And your tiredness vanishes just like that and you know it's all going to be ok.

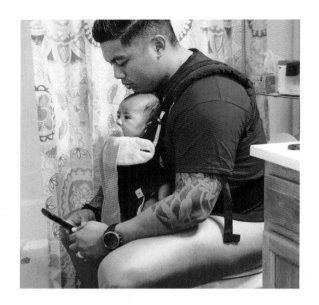

You'll become a
multi-tasking legend

Chestli Kris Buen @chestlikris

I was only 19 when I had my first baby, and I was fresh out of school ready to take on the world. I started to realise how difficult that could be when I wasn't able to get up and just go where I wanted and when I wanted. I had to start thinking about planning, finding sitters and what I could do if I had to stay home. It was a struggle at first. Everything changes down to your daily routine and you can't fight it.

What you can do is learn what things go together, and let go of what doesn't. It's hard to do something as simple as go to the bathroom in peace without a baby or toddler crying out for you, so why not just bring the baby? It's not a big deal. You can cook while the kids do homework, you can clean while they nap, you can all nap together (or clean together). You can squeeze in a few quick business calls or emails while your child is playing with their toys . . . I have a running stroller and bike trailer so my kids come out with me and enjoy a little ride, and sometimes they exercise too.

I know it's exhausting having to juggle multiple things at the same time. Sometimes, you're juggling your own sanity in that mix. But after you tuck the babies in and your head hits the pillow, you'll be proud that you kept yourself and the family together another day.

—— OUR ADVICE

Taking a dump with a baby on your lap might look or sound gross to the uninitiated but trust us when we say we've all done it! This super dad has taken it to the next level to free up his hands so he can keep up with his emails/do his online grocery shopping/text his mum back. What a dude!

No one tells you that when you become a parent you will automatically become a multi-tasking legend. We tell new parents that when they first change a shitty nappy it will be a two-handed or even two-person job, but after a while you'll find you can talk on the phone, purée carrots, put the washing away, wipe up poo, change a lightbulb and stop your baby from crying all at the same time!

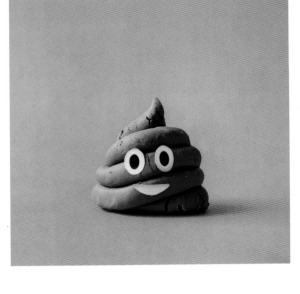

Sometimes it's shit

Rachel Sobel @whineandcheezits

I love being a mother with every fibre in my body but I don't understand why everyone is afraid to say how much it sucks as you try to rock a colicky baby to sleep at 2am when you really want to rock in a corner all by yourself. The admission does not mean you don't love your baby.

Can't we just be real about it? You know, like when someone asks, "OMG Susan! How's motherhood treating you?" instead of saying, "I've never been happier in my life," you say, "You know what, Carol? It's fucking miserable. Nobody in my house is sleeping. I can't get my shit together. My clothes are covered in bodily fluids that are not mine, and there isn't enough coffee on the planet right now."

ALSO:

- You're so sleep deprived that you actually start to feel like a three-hour stretch of sleep is the best thing to happen to you since the epidural
- You have no idea when you last showered
- Everything your partner says and does is pissing you off
- Actually, everything *anyone* says and does is pissing you off
- You have this brand new amazing life in your hands and all he/she does is cry, sleep, eat, poop, cry, poop, cry, eat, cry, cry, cry
- Even when the baby isn't crying, you still hear crying because you are slowly losing your mind

The first two months with a newborn are a shit-show. Figuratively. Literally. Hang in there.

—— OUR ADVICE

Those first few weeks can be so so hard, but do try and remember it will not always be like that. There may be days where you feel like you cannot take any more and you may doubt your ability to be a good parent. But the good news is that there will also be amazing days where you can't help but grin and thank your lucky stars for what you have. There will be days and nights where your baby sleeps like a dream, smiles and giggles and doesn't projectile poo, and those are the days that make it all feel worth it!

It's also good to know that not everyone finds it hard. Yes there really are people who breeze through these early days. They take to breastfeeding naturally and have a baby that feeds and sleeps and smiles. If this is you then that's wonderful, enjoy every moment and don't feel guilty about it.

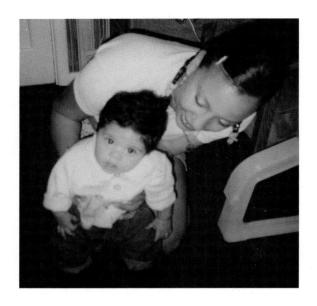

Having a baby at 18 does not mean your life is over

Marley Hall @midwifemarley
midwifemarley.com

Becoming a mother at 18 wasn't what I had planned. As with many young girls, I thought I would finish school, go to college, study for a degree and start a career before getting married and starting a family. All of those things happened, but in a completely different order.

I had my first baby at 18 while studying health and social care at college. I clearly recall giving birth in March and being back in lessons with my baby by April. My tutor was extremely accommodating and supportive as she wanted me to succeed as much as I did. The course finished in July and I was even given the award "student of the year 2000".

I never allowed myself to settle into the role of "just mum". I wanted more from life and after a stint at university, I became a midwife. Little did I know before that, while studying, there was actually quite a lot of support from the university with childcare. They gave me access to a fund that covered about 80% of my childcare costs.

Fast forward 20 years and I now have five children, the eldest being at university himself. I paved the way for my own opportunities and now I'm an experienced midwife and public speaker. Having a baby young has been challenging but not debilitating. I believe in always striving to be the best you possibly can with whatever life throws at you!

—— OUR ADVICE

Becoming a new mum is daunting, we can all agree on that! But for young mums it can be even harder. Being a young mum can sometimes be isolating and it may be difficult to meet other mums of a similar age. It can be upsetting to feel judged by others and this may knock your confidence. You may need financial support, especially if you have become a parent before establishing a career, and you may need extra guidance and help if you do not have good support networks in place. If you haven't yet gained experience with certain life skills, like cooking, budgeting, independence and personal development, then suddenly becoming responsible for another human being can be challenging.

Encouragement, making connections, meeting role models, educational support and training and access to employment are all things that can benefit younger mums who are struggling. Luckily there are lots of organisations out there that can help with this such as Home Start and The Young Mums Support Network.

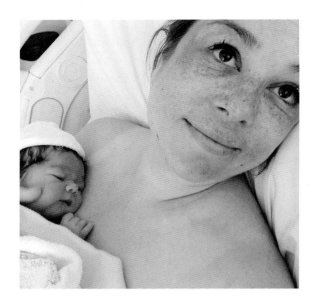

You will never shower
in peace again

Beth Willis @bethannawillis

You know that scene in *Mission: Impossible* where Tom Cruise
abseils down from the ceiling and the tension is absolutely heart-
pounding and a bead of sweat is about to fall off his head onto the
heat sensor alarm beneath him? Nobody tells you before you have
kids, that that will be you in the morning as you try and steal a few
moments in the shower alone.

In the pursuit of quiet, timing is everything. I will wait until they
are preoccupied with how much cereal they can share with the floor.
I will creep past them, nervously clutching my towel, with my internal

stopwatch already ticking dangerously low. They could not be less interested in conversation with me. And yet. Without fail, the minute the water hits me and the glorious sound of silence envelops me – I will open my eyes and there they will be. Like the twins from *The Shining*. Except grinning inanely and with unironed outfits, wanting a chat. "Why have you got a beard on your front bottom?" "Why are your boobies so long?" "Why don't you want to get a bunny rabbit?" "What does privacy mean?"

It's my fault of course. Those early, anxious days when you daren't let them out of your sight so you take them with you everywhere – including the bathroom. For them, the bathroom equals company and a good chat.

——— OUR ADVICE

When they are tiny you try to shower and they cry and your heart breaks and you have to jump out in a blind panic covered in soap, because you can't bear it any longer.

Then there is the toddler stage where they just thump on the shower door and scream while you wash your bits!

The next stage where they come and do a poo on the loo when you're in the shower and stink out the bathroom and then yell at you to get out and wipe their bum!

And then onto the stage where they might just set fire to the house or start playing with knives while you're in there!

It's important to know that a baby will not come to any harm if they are somewhere safe and cry for a few minutes while you wash yourself. You are not abandoning your child. You will not damage them psychologically or physically. There will always be times in your life when you cannot pick up your baby as soon as he or she cries and that is something that you will both learn to cope with. Don't worry.

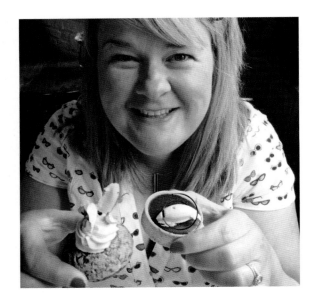

Self-care is so important

Mia O'Brien @be_more_cherry

Sadness crept in as I caught myself looking at my body and wondering why I no longer looked after it the way it deserved. When I was pregnant I nurtured it, cherished it, marvelled at its daily changes. There in the mirror was a mother, lost, disconnected from it, ignoring its needs. My body and mind had been seriously neglected.

Nobody ever told me self-care as a parent should be as important as feeding and caring for your baby. But with the help of family, friends and social media I realised that it needs to be seen as a necessity not a luxury.

Slowly self-care has filtered in, in many forms. The simplicity of switching to having a shower at night instead of the morning meant I could take my time. Telling myself it is ok to watch a favourite TV programme after bedtime rather than put away clean washing or read the latest nursery newsletter. It is ok to go to bed solo at 8pm so I can lie like a starfish, adorned with a warm soothing eye mask. It is ok to leave my little one in her bed a few extra minutes when she wakes so I can enjoy some precious sips of hot, reviving coffee. When working full-time I added in getting off the bus one stop earlier to have a brisk buggy-free walk. An episode of *Hey Duggee* in the morning meant I got to put my make-up on without having to share my eyeshadow brush with sticky porridge fingers.

A year on and we are both thriving. I tell myself that be it ten minutes, one hour, one day or even a few days – child-free time for me is absolutely ok!

—— OUR ADVICE

It's so true. We hope you all get some time out today to take care of yourself. If you can snatch a few minutes while your baby sleeps or your toddler plays (with a wooden puzzle or an iPad . . . we're not judging) don't feel bad about doing something for you whether that's a quick nap or a stretch or a cup of tea and some biscuits. Tidying the house can wait!

Self-care doesn't just drop out of the sky onto your lap. You need to be proactive about making preparations and arranging logistics so that you can find time to do something for yourself. It can feel strange and selfish to put yourself first, but the benefits should outweigh any doubts you might have about it.

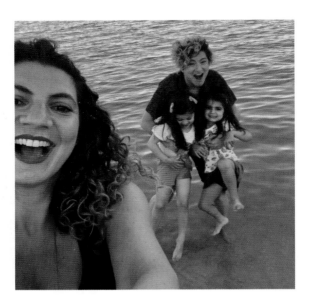

About being a same-sex parent

Jodie Lancet-Grant @jodielancetgrant
The Pirate Mums published by Oxford University Press, June 2021

I came out when I was 20. Nobody told me that having a baby (or in my case, twin babies) would mean doing it all over again.

In my pre-babies life, I didn't feel that the new people I met – at a bar, say, or a club or a house party – ever assumed anything about my sexuality. But in the almost uniformly single-sex environments of Baby Sensory, Baby Music Class and Baby Hartbeeps, that was not the case. Time and again I would see a (generally well and quickly concealed) look of surprise flit across a fellow mum's face when I mentioned my wife. And really, did it matter if the friendly woman I chatted to by the swings – and everyone else – assumed I was straight? In some ways, no. These relationships hardly went deep. But I was surprised by how heteronormative maternity leave felt, and how often I didn't feel like myself, being aware of the assumptions being made about me but knowing it would be weird to blurt out "ACTUALLY I'M MARRIED TO A WOMAN" during a low-key chat about sleep deprivation.

I don't blame any of these women for this. After all, there are precious few representations of families like mine in the stories we read to our kids, the TV shows we watch, or any of the media we consume. I hope my book, *The Pirate Mums*, starts to go some way to redress the balance.

—— OUR ADVICE

Becoming a new parent is taxing enough without the added pressure of worrying about what other people may think about your sexuality and how you are bringing up your children. Meeting other new parents is often a tricky and nerve-wracking process, and you may be particularly worried about the lack of understanding and support or insensitivity from potential new friends.

Explaining your own, unique relationship status and family make-up to new friends, teachers, doctors and even your own family members can sometimes feel daunting and difficult. Although the world has become a kinder and more understanding place in recent years, the lack of relevant examples in mainstream media means that many people have misconceptions about LGBTQIA+ people's ability to have children and to be great parents.

Let's help spread the message that your sexuality, or the way that your baby came to you, does not affect your ability to be a wonderful parent. It is up to us all to promote positivity and pride among all parents.

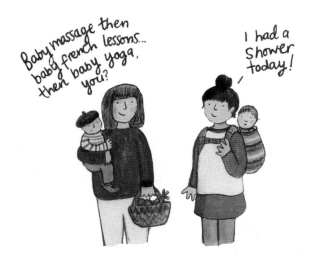

Some days it's about just surviving

Helene @helenetheillustrator
helenetheillustrator.co.uk

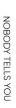

Nobody tells you it's ok if all you did today is survive! With a newborn baby every day is survival . . . You'll never enjoy shopping for bog roll on your own as much as at this point in your life. A trip to the supermarket alone can feel like a spa day!

A FEW THINGS I WISH SOMEONE HAD TOLD ME . . .
• Nobody knows what they're doing, we're all making this up as we go along and hoping for the best.

- If you have a shower today, it's a massive achievement, even if you can't relax in there.
- Try not to feel bad if you're not enjoying your new "role" – what kind of crazy person actually enjoys sleep deprivation, being shat on, having your nipples turn black and walking like John Wayne for weeks with not so much as a smile of thanks in return?
- If all you've done today is sit on the sofa and feed your baby, change shitty nappies and destroy a family-sized tin of biscuits . . . that's completely fine. Motherhood will bless you with endless opportunities to feel guilty, don't make these early days one of them. Just make sure you're set up with drinks, snacks and your phone in close proximity before you plonk your bum down.
- And most importantly: don't put so much pressure on yourself, and ignore any smug-faced mums who tell you their baby is sleeping through the night at two weeks old – it's most likely bullshit.

It's all worth it by the way. You'll blink and they'll be a stroppy four-year-old.

—— OUR ADVICE

There is a lot of pressure on women to look like they're "nailing it" when in fact most of us are just "winging it". Try not to compare yourself to others, because there will always be someone who looks like they're doing a better job than you today. We all have days where we feel like we are failing, and equally we have days where we think we have it all under control and are winning at this parenting lark. Try to celebrate the good days, and on the more difficult ones, give yourself permission to just relax and take it easy if you can.

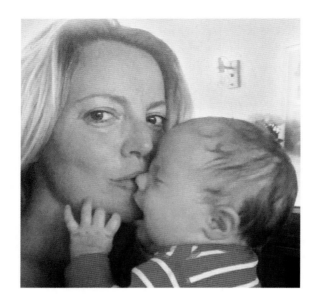

You will be so tired

Molly Gunn @selfishmother
SelfishMother.com

Nobody tells you that Saturday night would be spent shusshing
and jigging a restless bubba so much that by the time she finally
fell asleep I'd turn on Netflix to have some down time but I'd be so
exhausted that my eyes would start closing and I'd promptly fall
straight asleep too!

Everyone knows that babies don't always sleep well but
nobody tells you that once you have got them to sleep you don't
even have the energy to enjoy your time alone. Some days and
nights you can barely string a sentence together and yet you
are dying to do something with your down time – watch a movie,

catch up on the mounting queue of WhatsApp messages, or simply just sit down, and then before you know it your eyes are c...l...o...s...i...n...g and it's game over!

—— OUR ADVICE

It is so hard to explain to someone who doesn't yet have a baby how tired you get. Even people who are used to sleep deprivation – those who work night shifts or sleep four hours a night because of their demanding jobs are surprised about how hard it hits them in this newborn phase. It seems relentless and soul-destroying at times and you will often find yourself wondering how you can go on like this.

But don't worry: like all these things, it's just a phase (IT'S JUST A PHASE is a great mantra for new parents). Pretty soon your baby will be sleeping better and you will get a new lease of life! You may be forever slightly knackered but that's different to the complete and utter new mum exhaustion you feel at first.

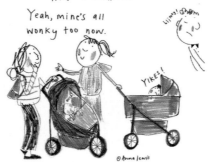

Only just met but ....

Yeah, so that bit is wonky now, oh that really wobbles and that bit blew up like a balloon!

Yeah, mine's all wonky too now.

Yikes!

© Anna Lewis

Oversharing becomes the norm

Anna Lewis @sketchymuma
annalewisstudio.co.uk

I am quite an open book anyway but it does make me chuckle how much you are willing to share with a perfect stranger after giving birth, while standing in the post office queue! I always found it a bit like speed dating in the early days, meeting new mums where you had about three minutes to connect before a nappy explosion or something and the chat was usually about your "birth story".

I suppose it is all so new having a baby and your body changes so much that you just want to feel normal, and sharing your experiences is a way of adjusting to your new body. It's actually pretty amazing what the human body does creating a baby, but it's comforting to know that other people were also sitting on a rubber ring for five days rather than out doing a 5k run a week after giving birth.

I remember having so many conversations in the early days at the playgroup about rips and tears and bodily fluids, but I don't really remember the specifics now of people's intimate body parts, which is reassuring! I think whatever stage of motherhood you are going through, conversations in general can be a lot more open and honest as we are all in it together.

—— OUR ADVICE

Nobody tells you what you will be willing to tell a perfect stranger after having a baby, but you might just find yourself chatting to other mums you just met about your fanny or your piles!

We're not sure what it is that compels new mums to want to share their most intimate details with someone they have just met in the supermarket, but it's true and it's great. How amazing to feel so at ease that talking about your fanny or bum with a complete stranger does not faze you! The relief when you meet someone who says, "YES, ME TOO!" is just huge and feels like a weight lifted. Whether it's a quick bitch about your partner, a chat about your episiotomy or how you wee yourself a bit when you sneeze, it can be very liberating! It's also great for helping to forge friendships as it helps you identify your people, the ones you can laugh and share your stories with.

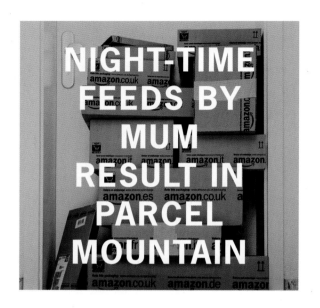

NIGHT-TIME FEEDS BY MUM RESULT IN PARCEL MOUNTAIN

About midnight spending sprees

Emma Harrison @canibreastfeedinituk
cibii.co.uk

Nobody tells you about the seemingly endless nights, the minimal amount of sleep, the feeding on demand, the being awake when the rest of the world sleeps. The long hours being awake, feeding all alone, just you and the baby in the dark of night.

And what is there to do when you can barely lift your tired eyelids? Reading sounds like a quality idea, but it is not easy when the sea of words blur into one . . . so how about a bit of retail therapy . . . Look at all those miracle baby items you have heard about, look at the "special offers", and they can all be delivered the next day!

And then you go back to sleep. The next day those night-time purchases are so quickly forgotten in that sleepy morning haze when you are somehow surviving on a few hours of interrupted shut-eye. Until a steady stream of parcels appears piled up at your door . . . a sure sign a new mum lives here!

—— OUR ADVICE

BEWARE! Anyone up with a non-sleeping baby in the middle of the night with a smartphone in their possession is in serious danger of hitting "BUY NOW". And you wake up bleary-eyed the next day to an Amazon Prime drone hovering outside your house delivering white-noise machines, special sleeping pods, expensive new-fangled swaddles and a whole host of other things that "customers who bought this item also bought" and you have a £300-sized hole in your bank account. And guess what? You'll be up again tonight wondering what else you can buy to try and get more sleep!

In this age of instant gratification and consumerism, it is tempting to reach for our wallets when faced with adversity. It is easy to jump to conclusions and assume that your crying baby is unhappy with its environment or the equipment you've bought. "He hates his Moses basket" is what we hear over and over. But it's not true. Your baby is too tiny to have an opinion about the brand of Moses basket he's lying in. He isn't pissed off because it's a hand-me-down one, he doesn't want you to go and buy a new one!

We're not saying there aren't some amazing products out there, and they may well help you and your baby get some more sleep, BUT do be aware of how susceptible you are to overspending at 2am. Wait until the morning before you make any bold purchasing decisions and think about things rationally in the light of day with a clearer head!

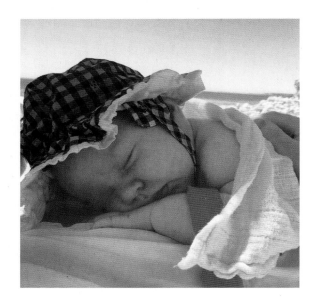

About routines

Ruth Ranson @ruth_ranson

Back when we were babies, there was one book (Dr Spock) and no internet. It must have been so much easier then . . . no bleary-eyed 3am Google searches, no perfect baby guides, no chirpy online experts telling you that you're doing it wrong.

   As each baby is different, so is each mum and their priorities and threshold levels. With my firstborn I wanted a routine and I wanted a manual, but which manual? Some of the preachy ones left me feeling really inadequate when I realised that I had failed dismally and it was only 8am and there were another 163 tasks to be fulfilled that day. The less direct ones weren't decisive enough for me. We tried them all. We did eventually find our rhythm and everyone was happy.

Our second born arrived seven years later. We had given up hope that there would even be a second born, so everything was different. Different baby, different priorities and different threshold levels.

I gave her the fourth trimester . . . why not? What's three more months when you've waited 84? I enjoyed the heck out of it but I was in a different state of mind and so decided that as long as I was getting enough sleep, I'd hold off dusting down the books or breaking out the searches.

And she slept well . . . until recently . . . recently the wheels kind of came off, but that's the thing about babies – they keep changing!

—— OUR ADVICE

Adults love a routine. Children love a routine. It gives them security and confidence when they know what is happening and when. Everyone needs routine to operate in the real world and if you want to go back to work at some stage you will need routine more than ever. But sometimes when we try and implement one too early it can cause more angst than peace.

Sure, there are things you can do to nudge your baby in the right direction and some take to it naturally more easily than others. Some babies sleep through the night from six weeks and some don't get it for a lot longer. But if you make sure they're getting the appropriate amount of sleep in the day for their age and persevere with the same bedtime and waking time every day, it will all fall into place eventually!

One important thing to note, though, is that you should not withhold feeds to try and push a routine into place as this doesn't always take growth spurts and your baby's need for comfort into account.

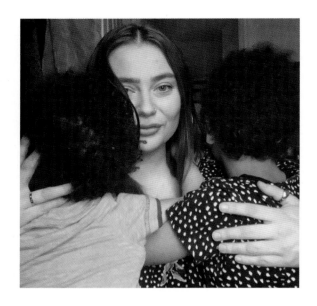

About being a single mum

Erin Smithers @erinmsmithers

noandroblog.com

It's easier! To clarify, it is easier to be a single mum than to be in an unproductive, toxic relationship. I started my motherhood as a single mum and I wouldn't be devastated if it ended as a single mum.

    I do wish I had someone to back me up on discipline, to do the school run when I'm unwell and to hold my hand when I've had a bad day. But actually, I have found greater support networks in friends: some mums, some not.

    The years I spent as part of a nuclear family unit were joyful at times too, but the stress, angst and anxieties that come with a less-than-ideal relationship were as time-consuming (if not more so) than the actual children who needed us to be solid.

As a single mum, it's likely that you'll cope with the really tough times on your own, as well as the mundane everyday parenting routine that can become monotonous and all-consuming. But you are also incredibly lucky to soak up all of the good to yourself, and you will be so proud of yourself when you realise what a good little egg you are raising and that it was all YOU. You did that!

—— OUR ADVICE

Whether becoming a single parent is a choice or the result of circumstances beyond your control, it can feel really overwhelming at times. Raising children alone, with no support from a partner, is relentless and your own mental and physical health may end up taking a back seat. It can also feel exhausting as you try to juggle childcare, a job and all the other mundane chores that make up everyday life. You may find yourself struggling financially, which can of course have a huge impact on you emotionally.

It is so important to try and find some support, whether from family, friends, charities, local organisations or other single parents. Charities like Gingerbread can help to put you in touch with other single parents in your area, which can be invaluable for things like swapping babysitting, lending a hand or even just someone to talk to who understands what you are going through. There is financial support available for you in the form of benefits, tax credits and child maintenance. Gingerbread can also help you with this side of things too.

Even though you may sometimes feel it, you are never alone. There is lots of help out there for you.

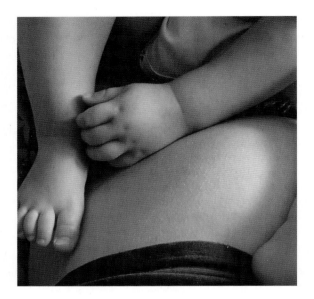

Parenting can be monotonous

Emily Elington @wildonesandme

Nobody tells you that parenting can sometimes feel isolating and monotonous. Sure they told me about the sleepless nights with a newborn baby but they didn't tell me about the sometimes mind-numbing exhaustion that comes from raising a feisty toddler.

Add pregnancy and a partner that works away a lot into that mix, not to mention a house move and general life upheaval, and I found myself recently going through the actions and routines that need doing without feeling part of them.

Keeping the small human alive and counting down till bedtime to do it all over again tomorrow. I don't feel like you have to be diagnosed with depression (or postnatal depression) to feel like this sometimes, but it sure can make you feel like a crappy parent. But I am trying, and I have started to get into more groups again and most importantly I am recognising the fact that I have been feeling totally drained. It comes down to that phrase again: "You can't pour from an empty cup." We all need some down time and time to ourselves. I just want other parents out there to know they are not alone if they have days where they just don't want to parent any more . . . It's ok. It's ok not to love every second as long as you love some of them. Nobody told me all this, but if you are struggling you are not alone.

───── OUR ADVICE

It can be so bloody monotonous and boring doing the same thing over and over again and you can spend every day counting down to the weekend (which is pretty similar to the week actually!). Feeding, nappies, cleaning, washing, folding, packing for leaving the house, feeding again, nappies again, supermarket, cooking, bathing, rocking and repeat! It can start to feel like Groundhog Day. Babies and small children are not known for showing their appreciation for all your hard work, so it can often feel a bit thankless and drudge-like. But hang on in there – there are lots of good days too. Hopefully today will be one of them!

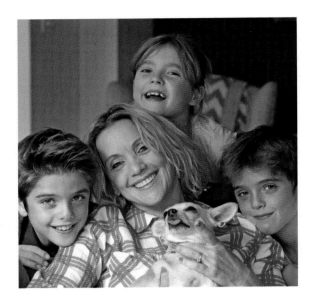

About coping with cancer and kids

Emma Campbell @limitless_em
All That Followed published by Mirror Books, 2018

Nobody tells you that the thing you longed for most in the world will sometimes bring with it the most enormous and unforeseen challenges. I was a newly single mum when I was diagnosed with breast cancer in 2010. My triplets were six months old and their big brother was nearly seven. After years of secondary infertility and recurrent miscarriage, it felt like the universe was playing the cruellest trick on us all. Those early weeks and months were a blur of night feeds, nappy changes and back-breaking trips up and down the stairs of our top-floor flat alongside chemotherapy, a mastectomy and radiotherapy. I was scared I wasn't bonding. I envied other mums who spoke of "pulling up the drawbridge" to fully embrace those early days while I passed my babies from person to person and wept as my hair fell out. I felt cheated of the luxury of peace of mind, of cherishing every second with the babies I'd spent years wishing into being.

But that was then. I am here and doing well. My "babies" are ten now, my big boy nearly 17. We are a noisy, messy, door-slamming, perfectly imperfect family – and for that I am so, so grateful.

—— OUR ADVICE
Being unwell can change everything. Instead of being able to focus on your new baby and your new role, you may find yourself consumed with your health issues and unable to enjoy this special time. Appointments, treatments and medication may become part of everyday life, as well as tiredness, pain, sickness and often complete mental and physical exhaustion.

Your loved ones will be worried too. They may not know how to talk to you or what to do. Being unwell may impact some of your close relationships and you may feel isolated or misunderstood at times. Try to keep communication going surrounding your illness. Talking openly may help those around you to feel able to do the same. Do not be afraid to accept support, or to let people know if help is not needed.

Although it is often easier said than done, try to maintain some sense of normality. Accept social invitations and try to stay in touch with the people who make you laugh and feel good. You are still the same person you were before.

If you need support with employment, financial or psychological issues, or advice about talking about your illness, there are some amazing organisations out there that can help: Home Start and Mummy's Star are great places to start.

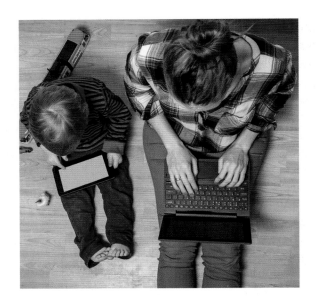

If you should go back to work or not

Lou Hake @louhake

Nobody ever told me I might want to be a stay-at-home mum.
I'm ashamed to admit that before I had my daughter, I thought
it looked like the easy option. How wrong I was!

    If you'd told me at any point during the first three months that
I'd choose not to go back to my job, I'd never have believed you.
I remember trying to rock my baby to sleep, furious at the mindless
monotony of it, physically exhausted by the feeding and sleep
deprivation. I really struggled with the transition to motherhood.
I was not prepared.

But then something changed. I started to enjoy it. Even when I feel like I've done a whole day by 9am or the final push to bedtime feels like it's going to break you, there is something so raw about raising your child.

My high-pressure, high-stress job had always defined me. But as the end of my maternity leave approached, I knew I wasn't ready to go back to work.

Financially this is not something we planned for but while my savings last, I want to dedicate this time to raising my daughter. I feel so privileged to have the opportunity to watch her little personality emerge and play whatever part I can.

I am starting to feel the "pull" of working so am looking for a part-time job, but it will have to be something that works around our family.

—— OUR ADVICE

Women go back to work after having babies for so many reasons, and one thing that's for sure is that it isn't a decision that's made lightly. You may work because you need to, financially or psychologically. You may work because you want to, to pay for holidays or private schools. You may work because your career is your passion and because without it, you don't feel like you.

Equally, if you have decided to stay at home with your baby, because you want to or you need to, then you don't need to justify this to anyone. Whether you work or don't work, whether it's you or a childminder who gives your baby lunch, whether your little one takes his or her lunchtime nap at home or at nursery, it doesn't matter – as long as you are happy with the decision and it works for you and your family.

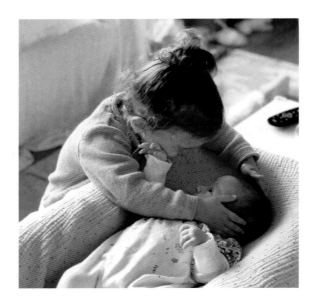

About having another baby

Natalia Sarah @newmummyadventures

Nobody tells you that even if you've always dreamt of giving your firstborn a sibling, the guilt you experience in your second pregnancy can be pretty consuming. Ava was 14 months old when I fell pregnant. Initially wrapped up in a bubble of excitement, I found that as the sickness and tiredness struck me, so did feelings of guilt and anxiety.

We'd made a decision that would change the world as Ava knew it – precious moments between just the two of us would be limited, the mummy/firstborn dynamic forever altered. And could I even love another baby the way I loved Ava?

Although my feelings were part of the emotional transition

of becoming a family of four, the guilt and worry were intense at the time. Then Alyssa arrived. I thought I knew pure joy, but the first time I saw Ava kiss Alyssa, my heart felt like it might actually explode. I worried Ava's world would be turned upside down, but she doesn't remember life without her pint-sized little bestie, who she absolutely adores. Don't get me wrong, there were times, especially in the first few weeks/months, when I felt I was treading water and failing them both. But those moments pass, and very quickly it feels like you didn't "change" anything at all, you just added in your missing piece.

—— OUR ADVICE

There is no right or wrong time to add to your family, and indeed there is no pressure to add to it at all if you don't want to. But you shouldn't worry too much about your child adapting to a new sibling. Little children are so resilient and usually adjust so easily to the addition of a baby to the house. Even if it does take a while for your first child to adapt, which sometimes happens, especially if they are a little older when their sibling arrives, this is usually a phase and nothing to be too worried about. You might feel emotional about the new baby being born as it marks the end of your time alone with your firstborn, but it is the start of a new chapter for your family and it is absolutely breathtaking to watch them learn to love and interact with their new brother or sister.

As for the timing of this second baby, well of course it's up to you and Mother Nature, but it is a good idea to wait at least a year before conceiving again. The "fourth trimester" can last longer than you might expect and you need time to adjust to the physical and psychological changes you have been through before starting again.

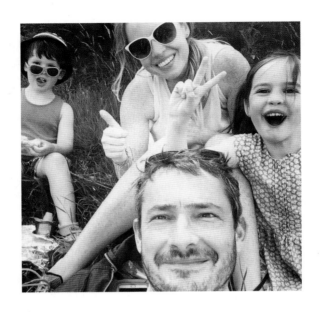

You are meant to know all the answers

Esther Coren @onthespike
onthespike.com

Nobody tells you that you are expected to have ALL the answers! People talk a load of shit about how you "find your own way" but from the minute the baby is born there are all these eyes looking at you expectantly – like, what do you wanna do now?

Sure you can be a strict routine queen or you can be a relaxed hippy but what if you just DON'T KNOW?

What if you don't know whether to try harder with breastfeeding or to give up? What if you don't know if it's teething or a cold? What if you don't know whether pink on girls is sexist or not? What if you don't know if you should go to A&E or not? How do you know what a tiny baby or a screeching toddler or even a stressed-out four-year-old really wants or needs?

I'm used to it now. I'm the freaking sergeant major SAS captain, Oracle of Delphi, Ceefax and Google of this damned house. And that's ok I suppose.

But at first, the realisation that THIS is what responsibility is . . . that was a shock!

——— OUR ADVICE
No matter how many books you read or classes you attend, when that baby pops out you are suddenly in charge of a whole new life and you need to start making decisions! And it's true, we don't always know if we're making the right choices. Some choices feel monumental (like how to react to that rash) and some choices feel tiny (apple rice cake or carrot stix) but someone needs to step up, and guess what? It's you! Be confident and trust your intuition – and don't do too much googling!

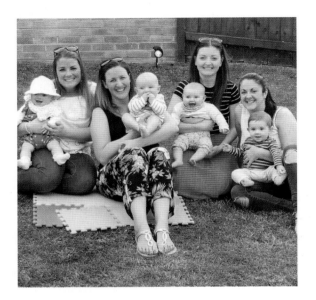

New mum friends are amazing

Sian Dando @12pawsandababy
spuddedando.wixsite.com/12pawsandababy

Your "mum friends" are more than just friends. They're your people, your village, your safety net, your besties.

When I was pregnant, I embarked on a mission to bag myself some "mum friends". I found myself at yoga and antenatal classes trying to find any little reason to swap numbers with other mums-to-be. I may as well have been jumping with my hands up shouting, "Please be my friend!"

But this is the best thing I ever did, as I ended up finding my tribe. Starting off as an awkward messaging group, it became our go-to for any baby questions and the place to be at 2am. Receiving that first "I'm awake too!" felt like a virtual hug, and suddenly I wasn't alone. These women soon became the people I felt (and still feel) lost without speaking to every day.

They've smiled with me through the good times, hugged me through the hard times, listened non-judgementally to my mummy fails, shared sweaty boob jokes with me, provided tea and cake, joined in with a much-needed lunchtime G&T, and laughed with me when there's nothing left to do but laugh.

They're more than mum friends; they've helped to define my new life as a parent and shape me to be the mum I am today. Now these amazing little people will keep us on this rollercoaster journey together for years to come. Here's to watching our babies grow up together!

——— OUR ADVICE

You really might make new friends that you will come to love as much as your old ones! Chance meetings in the nappy aisle in the supermarket, at Rhyme Time in the library, at baby weigh-in or while looking round a nursery, might be the key to your new mum gang.

And what about your online friends? It sounds so odd to think of these people that you only know by their @name as being your friends. But there are some incredibly supportive people out there on Facebook and Instagram and even though you may never meet them, it's good to know they've got your back.

If you have ever benefited from the support or shoulder of a friend, you'll know how amazing it can be, so try and make sure you pay it forward. Be that friend to someone else. Give a new parent a ring or a text today and see if they are ok, plan a visit or just have a chat.

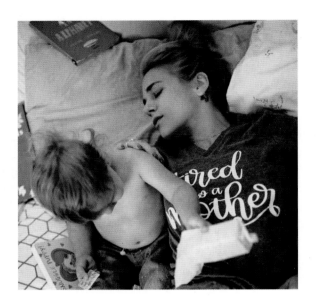

There would be days like these

Lauren Archer @loveofalittleone
loveofalittleone.com

Nobody tells you that some days it feels like too much. It doesn't feel worth it and you just can't take much more.

I did not want to mom today.

This noun-turned-verb exhausts me. There were no naps, no moments of quiet. Your exploratory side which seemed so cute just yesterday is now more of a solid annoyance.

Today has been filled with wasted time. Time spent cooking food you didn't eat. Time spent dressing you in clothes you destroyed. Time spent cleaning messes – careless, frivolous, foreseen messes. Time spent daydreaming about when two was one and I was free to do things without first mapping out the logistics of naps and snacks and how much you hate the car.

There was laughter and joy, yes, but today the scales never evened out and those moments just didn't make it worth it. Was that horrible to say? It's the truth. I would have traded your laughter for being able to sleep in, to drink my coffee while it was still warm, for a little bit of slack on the chain that tethered me to you today.

Today ended in tears, mine not yours. You were too busy jumping on me, pulling me, not understanding that I am human too. That my body hurts, my mind is shot, my spirit low. I forget I deserve respect and understanding and a little bit of space.

So I give in, that feeling of worthlessness creeping in, hand in hand with guilt.

Is this what being a shitty mom feels like? Or is this what moms just feel like on a shitty day?

—— OUR ADVICE

It is absolutely ok to have days like these. This does not make you a bad mother. Every parent has days where they feel like packing it all in. Keeping another human alive is relentless and sometimes not as rewarding as you may think. It can feel like a thankless task as you complete mundane chores and plod from one day to the next. You may not get the mental or physical space you feel you need and this can be very difficult.

But please understand this won't be forever. The good days are always just around the corner. The hugs, kisses, smiles, giggles and milestones will help you along the way. In the meantime, try and take time out to do something for yourself. Try mindfulness, yoga, walking, running, sleeping, reading, socialising or even just a few minutes alone in peace, with your own thoughts.

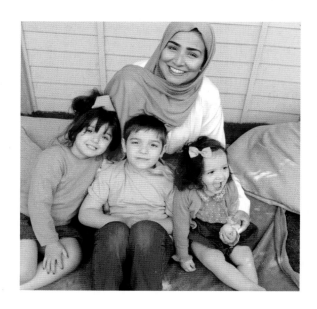

About being a Muslim mum

Nilly Dahlia @Nillydahlia

Being the only brown Muslim in a predominantly white middle-class village, I was never approached, never smiled at nor acknowledged at baby groups. I went to a number of groups to find like-minded mothers, but I was invisible. This is when it hit me how lonely motherhood can be. I see so many new mothers having coffee dates with other new mothers that they became friends with from their antenatal classes and I never had that.

This is what unconscious bias looks like. They were conditioned to believe being white is superior and holds the most power. You only have to look at many mummy friend circles to see this. Being a brown Muslim means I didn't fit in because society has conditioned white people to believe I am less than them. This makes me sad.

Without realising, society has trained people to believe that Muslims are "terrorists", "oppressed", "radical" and "towelheads" – and they wouldn't want a friend like that. They make their assumptions of me from what the media has portrayed, so I was never given a chance. But when I became a mother, I realised how much more important it is for our circles to be wide and for our children to be friends with a large variety of people. You are not born racist. It is something that is taught, even subconsciously. If you went through your child's bookshelf, how many books have non-white characters? Probably not many. As parents we need to raise our children better. We need for them to see all of the kids in the room and treat everyone as their equal. Maybe this way, society's perception of Muslims will finally change.

—— OUR ADVICE

It is so common for new parents to feel isolated. Even if you attend a baby group where the other new mums look like you, it is not unusual to feel you don't fit in. This is much more pronounced when your skin is a different colour or you wear traditional dress.

It is our duty as new parents to instil an anti-racist mindset in our children. Education starts at home and it is never too early to start talking to your children about race. It is never too early to teach your children to treat all human beings with respect and kindness. It is never too late to educate yourself and to edit your children's toys and books to include more diversity.

Try to lead by example and reach out to that mum who is sitting alone. She might not look like you, but she speaks the universal language of motherhood! She is going through the same stuff as you: the cracked nipples and the sleepless nights. She worries about the same things as you.

Make motherhood a force for good – take this chance to make connections, build relationships and broaden your own horizons and those of your children.

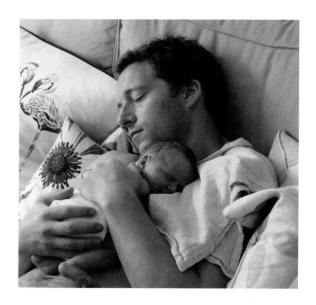

About becoming a dad

Tom Maberly @mrwhitetv
mrwhite.tv

Nobody ever tells you to enjoy the period of feeling on cloud nine! There has been nothing like it for me, the pride I felt when I held my babies for the first time, the love you feel for your partner for having got through this monumental feat – the conclusion being the most beautiful, perfect human being in your forever-changed world.

You hear so much about sleepless nights and the loss of your "old life", but there was a period of such utter joy and exhilaration in the immediate aftermath of both our children's births that I felt like I was living on a different planet. If you could bottle that feeling it would be some medicine!

It's impossible to feel absolutely, comprehensively ready, both practically and mentally, but the key for me was, and continues to be, to keep an open mind and roll with the punches. The emotional rollercoaster is exciting and all-consuming, and the pleasure of creating and helping to manage the newly expanded unit that your newborns fill is an honour and a privilege that I will never take for granted. It's a role I wholeheartedly signed up for, and is worth it more than I could have ever comprehended.

—— OUR ADVICE

The partners often get overlooked in the excitement of the arrival of a new baby. Praise and advice is heaped on the new mother and every other iota of attention is saved for cooing over the baby.

We sometimes forget that everything has changed for our partners too. Their emotions and their needs usually take a back seat in the early days. Perhaps this is because their contribution to this whole journey has until this moment, for obvious reasons, been limited! But let's give the other parents their moments too. Let them hold their baby without breathing down their neck. Let them learn to parent, just as you are. We are all winging it, so isn't it wonderful to have a wingman or woman!

A poem for you

May your coffee be strong

May your standards be realistic

May your inner voice be kind

May you replace perfection with "enough"

May you devour the fun moments

And breathe through the tough ones

May you cut many corners

And then,

As the eve draws near,

May your sofa be spacious and comfy,
for flopping

Anna Mathur @annamathur

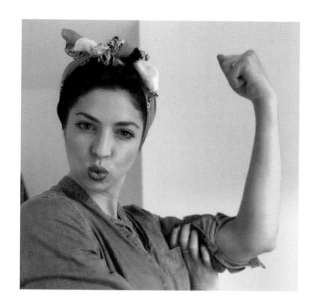

You can do it!

Anna Mathur @annamathur
annamathur.com

Feast on the good moments like an all-you-can-eat buffet. Gulp them down like an ice-cold can of Coke on a hot day. Etch the memories across every inch of your heart like a mosaic of tattoos. Man they're good. Smile until your cheeks ache, marvel at the fact you made them. Your heart swells, and your ability to juggle increases.

And you discover strengths and depths to yourself that you didn't know existed. You never knew you'd be able to endure the challenges you have, function on the little sleep you've had. You never would have considered that you could find someone so

NOBODY TELLS YOU

delicious you were genuinely concerned you may eat them.

What about the not-so-good moments? It's ok not to enjoy them. Take deep breaths, roar like a lioness behind a closed door. Wish the hour to fly, hunger for bedtime. Text a friend from the kitchen floor. Grab your lifelines. Exercise the muscle of vulnerability. You are absolutely worthy of the care and support you offer others, and accepting it is a strength worth learning and teaching.

Accept the gestures, the hugs, and the kind words. Let them hold you up as you swerve through those days caffeine fuelled and sleep deprived. Oh, your feelings are so valid. However acceptable or not you deem them to be, don't devalue or diminish them by comparing them with what you see of someone else's experience.

Motherhood is hard and great. It's exhausting and invigorating. And you want time to both slow and speed up. And you're thriving and surviving and enduring and being challenged and changed and all the things, and all the feelings. And that's ok. You're allowed to feel many things at once. How you feel in any moment is neither a reflection of how much you love your child or how good a parent you are. The feelings will recede like the tide. Ride them.

And for those moments where you cry, "I can't do this!": you can. Because, well, look: you are! And you have. And you will do again.

You are doing it

Nobody needs to tell you this. You know it yourself. But we are here to remind you. You *are* doing it . . .

From the moment you watch those little blue lines appear, see that heart beating on the scan, and dare to dream of names and wonder what they might look like.

As you battle the aches and pains and nerves of the first trimester, moan and groan your way through that last trimester.

From the moment you feel that first contraction or are wheeled into the operating theatre, when you put your nerves aside and concentrate on the task of giving birth to your baby.

When you first set eyes on their scrunched-up little red face and hear their little voice and hold them in your arms.

On the days that feel so rotten that it is only when they are finally asleep that you can breathe easily, and you head to bed defeated and guilt-stricken.

On the days that feel so incredible that you will want to give yourself a medal and shout from the rooftops about what a great parent you are.

You can do it.

289

For more detailed info on anything you have read, please check out our website & online antenatal classes at **amotherplace.com** and join our supportive community on social media **@amotherplace.**

BABY SUPPLIES & GENERAL SUPPORT

Home Start home-start.org.uk
Little Village littlevillagehq.org
Baby banks like this provide free vital baby supplies for those in need. A map of baby banks across the UK can be found at littlevillagehq.org/uk-baby-banks

BIRTH TRAUMA

The Birth Trauma Association birthtraumaassociation.org.uk
Make Birth Better @birthbetter

BOTTLE FEEDING

Don't Judge Just Feed dontjudgejustfeed.com
NHS UK nhs.uk/conditions/pregnancy-and-baby/bottle-feeding-advice
Unicef unicef.org.uk

BREASTFEEDING

Analytical Armadillo analyticalarmadillo.co.uk
The Breastfeeding Network breastfeedingnetwork.org.uk
Lactation Consultants of Great Britain lcgb.org
La Leche laleche.org.uk
Kelly Mom kellymom.com

CANCER

Mummy's Star mummysstar.org

COLIC & REFLUX

Living with Reflux livingwithreflux.org
NHS nhs.uk/conditions/reflux-in-babies
The Parent and Baby Coach theparentandbabycoach.com

CO-SLEEPING

Baby Sleep Info Source (BASIS) basisonline.org.uk

UNICEF unicef.org.uk/
babyfriendly/baby-friendly-
resources/sleep-and-night-time-
resources/caring-for-your-baby-
at-night
Lullaby Trust lullabytrust.org.uk

and, if possible, respond by
coughing or tapping the headset.
Or call 999 from a mobile and when
prompted just dial 55 and you will
be connected to the police, who will
know you are not able to speak.

DEPRESSION & ANXIETY
During or after pregnancy
APNI apni.org | 0207 386 0868
Hub of hope hubofhope.co.uk
Mind mind.org.uk | 0300 123 3393
PANDAS pandasfoundation.org.uk
0808 1961 776
Samaritans Samaritans.org | 116 123

Call 999 if it is an emergency

Supporting men
Andys Man Club @andysmanclubuk
The Dad's Network thedadsnet.com

HYPEREMESIS GRAVIDARUM
Pregnancy Sickness Support
pregnancysicknesssupport.org.uk
Search Instagram for the
hashtags #hyperemesis
#hyperemesisgravidarum
#pregnancysicknesssupport

HYPNOBIRTHING
Natal Hypnotherapy
natalhypnotherapy.co.uk
The Positive Birth Company
@thepositivebirthcompany

DOMESTIC ABUSE
**The National Domestic
Abuse Helpline**
nationaldahelpline.org.uk
**Freephone 24-hr for confidential
support: 0808 2000 247**

**If you are in danger and unable to
talk on the phone, call 999 and listen
to the questions from the operator**

INFERTILITY
Big Fat Negative @bigfatnegative
Infertility Illustrated
@infertilityillustrated
IVF Babble @ivfbabble
IVF Explained @ivf_explained
Search Instagram for hashtags
#ttc #ivf #ivfsupport #transferday
#eggcollection #ivfcycle

MAKING FRIENDS

Mummy Buddy @mummy_buddy
Mummy Social @mummysocial
Mush @mushmums
Peanut @peanut

MISCARRIAGE & LOSS

The Ectopic Pregnancy Trust
ectopic.org.uk
I Had a Miscarriage
@ihadamiscarriage
Lullaby Trust lullabytrust.org.uk
The Miscarriage Association
miscarriageassociation.org.uk
Sands sands.org.uk
Spring springsupport.org.uk
Tommy's @tommys

PELVIC FLOOR

Jane Wake @janewakeuk
Mothers Wellness Toolkit
@mothers.wellness.toolkit
The Mummy Coach
@themummycoach.co.uk
Physio Mum @physiomumuk
Umi Health @umihealth

POSTPARTUM PSYCHOSIS

Action on Postpartum Psychosis
app-network.org

PREMATURE BABY

Bliss bliss.org.uk
March of Dimes marchofdimes.org
Tommy's tommys.org
Twins Trust twinstrust.org

SAME-SEX PARENT SUPPORT

Donor Conception Network
dcnetwork.org
Some Families podcast
play.acast.com/s/somefamilies
Stonewall stonewall.org.uk
We Are Family magazine
wearefamilymagazine.co.uk

SINGLE PARENT SUPPORT

Citizens Advice citizensadvice.org.uk
Gingerbread gingerbread.org.uk

WORK/MATERNITY RIGHTS

Government services gov.uk
Maternity Action
maternityaction.org.uk
Mother Pukka @mother_pukka
Pregnant Then Screwed
@pregnant_then_screwed

YOUNG MUMS

Home Start home-start.org.uk
Young Mums Support Network
ymsn.co.uk

———— PICTURE CREDITS

Copyright in the photographs and images used throughout this book remain the property of the contributors who supplied the photographs and images that accompany their story. The ownership of each work can be identified by the personal name attached to each story, with the exception of the following images: **Pg 58:** Malvestida Magazine on Unsplash | **Pg 63:** Collins Lesulie on Unsplash | **Pg 79:** Siobhan Miller @thepositivebirthcompany | **Pg 80:** Wenping Wang on Unsplash | **Pg 99:** Abi Roberts | **Pg 128:** Madison Ralg on Unsplash | **Pg 192:** Jernej Graj on Unsplash

—— ACKNOWLEDGEMENTS

This book has been a team effort and I am so lucky to have had access to so much expert advice and support from not only friends and family, but also the amazing community we are proud to call A Mother Place. Thank you to:

My father, **Roger Marwood**, for instilling in me my fascination with all things pregnancy and birth, and for providing his expert advice for this book.

My mother, **Suzie Marwood**, for casting her beady eyes over every word and always providing constructive criticism and enthusiasm.

My sister, **Sophie Constable**, for always being a great sounding board and telling me straight up if it was crap!

My brother, **Joe Marwood,** for his support from down under.

Our designer, **Danii Kedik,** for her patience and expertise.

Our proofreader, **Amber Burlinson**, for seeking out all the typos!

Anna Erwin-Iles for her help in getting the book to print.

Mandie Gower for giving me her excellent opinion on so many aspects of the book.

Photographer **Emilie Sandy** for kindly offering to take the authors' portraits.

Our **Kickstarter supporters** for believing in the idea and helping fund the first 2,000 copies.

My agent **Clare Hulton** for making this happen so smoothly.

Martha Burley, Baby Jack, Isabel Hewitt and the team at Bluebird.

Everyone who has shared their stories and photos with us. We could not have done this without you!

My husband, **Tom Maberly**, for your positivity and encouragement and for constantly telling me I could do it. You were right, I did do it! Thank you for being my biggest supporter, and the best father and husband I could imagine.

——— INDEX

This edition published 2021 by Bluebird
an imprint of Pan Macmillan
The Smithson, 6 Briset Street, London EC1M 5NR
Associated companies throughout the world
www.panmacmillan.com
EU representative: Macmillan Publishers Ireland Limited,
Mallard Lodge, Lansdowne Village, Dublin 4

ISBN 978-1-5290-5605-1

135798642
A CIP catalogue record for this book is available from the British Library.
Printed and bound in China

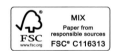

Interior design by kedikcreative.com

The information provided in this book is not an alternative to medical advice from your doctor or other professional healthcare provider. You should not delay in seeking medical advice, disregard medical advice or discontinue any medical treatment because of any information provided in this book. If you are worried or have any questions about any pregnancy-related or other medical matter then please consult your healthcare provider.

We are aware that not all family units have a male and female parent, but when it comes to the use of titles and pronouns we have used "mum", "mother", "dad", "father", "he" and "she" for brevity.

Every effort has been made to trace the copyright holders and obtain permission to reproduce this material. Please get in touch with any enquiries or any information relating to photographs or other content that appear in this Work.

So far as the author is aware the information given is correct and up to date as at October 2020. Practice, laws and regulations all change and the reader should obtain up to date professional advice on any such issue. The authors and publishers do not assume and disclaim, as far as the law allows, any liability to any party arising directly or indirectly from the use, or misuse, of the information contained in this book, or for any loss, damage, or disruption caused by errors or omissions, whether such errors or omissions result from negligence, accident, or any other cause.

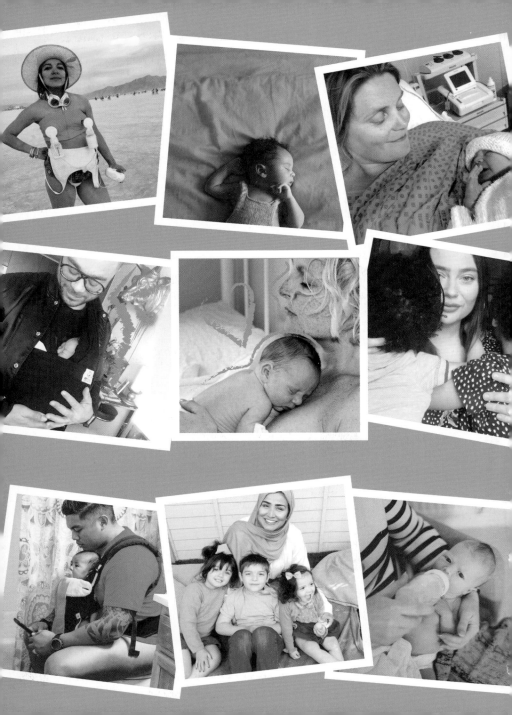